Oral Physiology

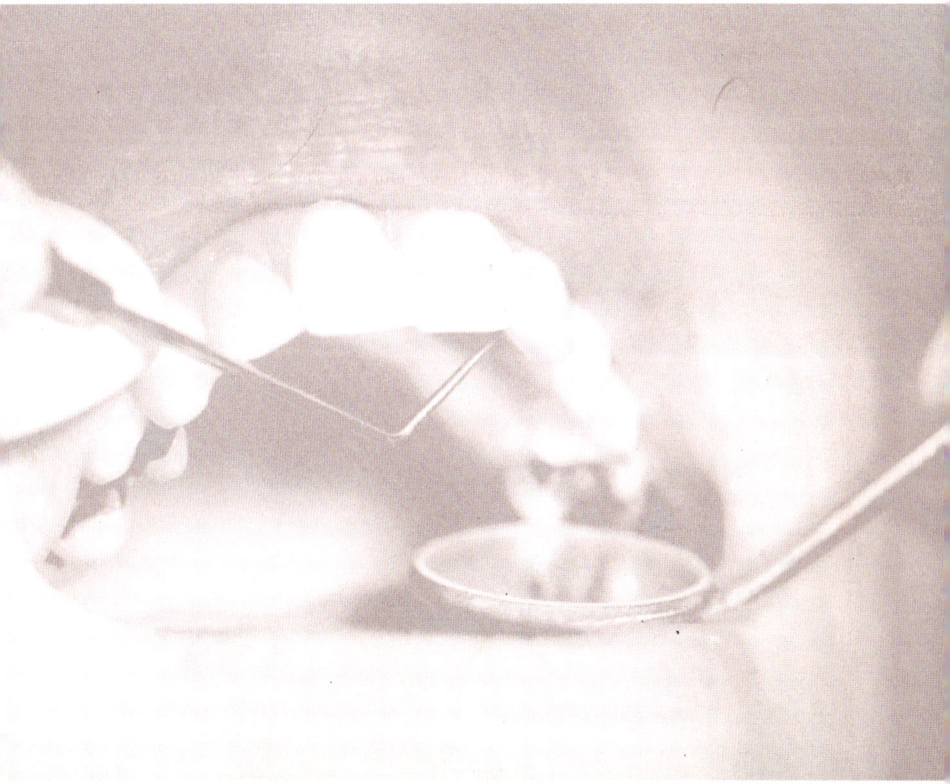

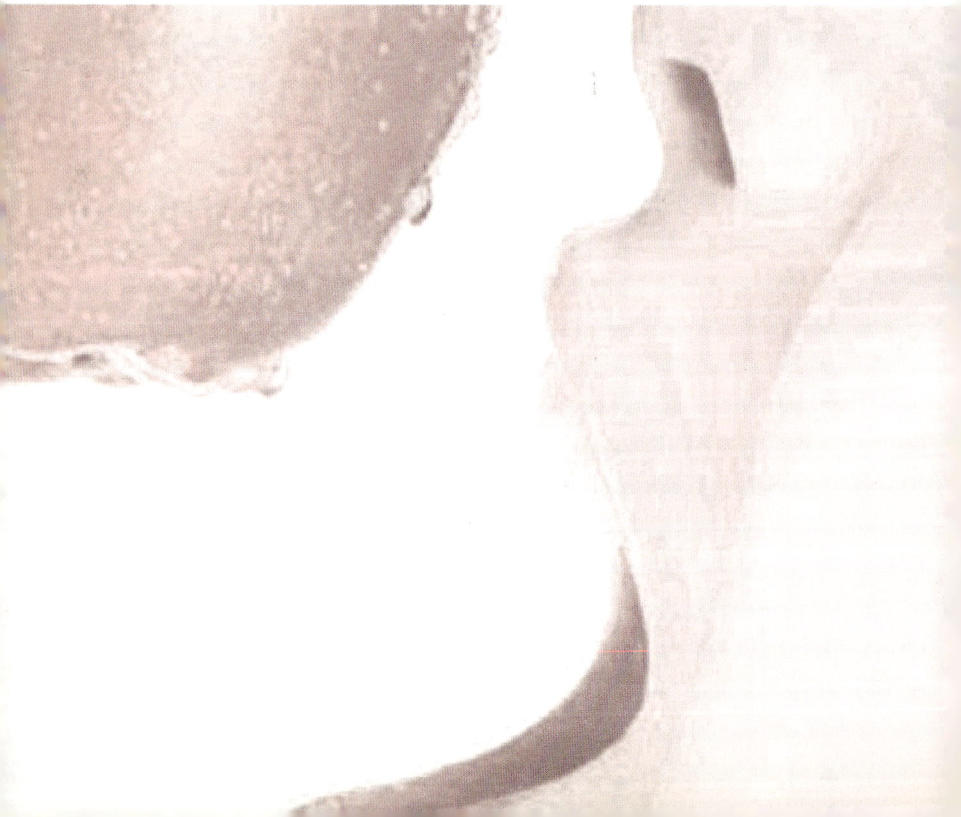

Oral Physiology

Shailja Chatterjee MDS, FAGE

Assistant Professor
Department of Oral and Maxillofacial Pathology
MM College of Dental Sciences and Research
Maharishi Markandeshwar University
Mullana-Ambala
Haryana

CBS

CBS Publishers & Distributors Pvt Ltd

New Delhi • Bengaluru • Pune • Kochi • Chennai

Oral Physiology

First Edition: 2011

ISBN: 978-81-239-1931-7

Published by Satish Kumar Jain and produced by Vinod K. Jain for

CBS Publishers & Distributors Pvt Ltd

Head off: CBS Plaza, 4819/XI Prahlad Street, 24 Ansari Road, Daryaganj, New Delhi 110 002, India

Ph: 23289259, 23266861/67 Website: **www.cbspd.com** Fax: +91-11-23243014 e-mail: delhi@cbspd.com cbspubs@vsnl.com cbspubs@airtelmail.in

Branches

- Bengaluru: Seema House 2975, 17th Cross, K.R. Road, Banasankari 2nd Stage, Bengaluru 560 070, Karnataka
  Ph: +91-80-26771678/79 Fax: +91-80-26771680 e-mail: bangalore@cbspd.com
- Pune: Bhuruk Prestige, Sr. No. 52/12/2+1+3/2 Narhe, Haveli (Near Katraj-Dehu Road Bypass), Pune 411 051, Maharashtra
  Ph: 020-64704058-59, 32342277 Fax: +91-020-24300160 e-mail: pune@cbspd.com
- Kochi: 36/14 Kalluvilakam, Lissie Hospital Road, Kochi 682 018, Kerala
  Ph: +91-484-4059061-65 Fax: +91-484-4059065 e-mail: cochin@cbspd.com
- Chennai: 20, West Park Road, Shenoy Nagar, Chennai 600 030, Tamil Nadu
  Ph: +91-44-26260666, 26208620 Fax: +91-44-45530020 email: chennai@cbspd.com

Printed at Paras Offset Pvt. Ltd., C-176, Naraina Industrial Area Phase-I, New Delhi

to

my family

and

teachers

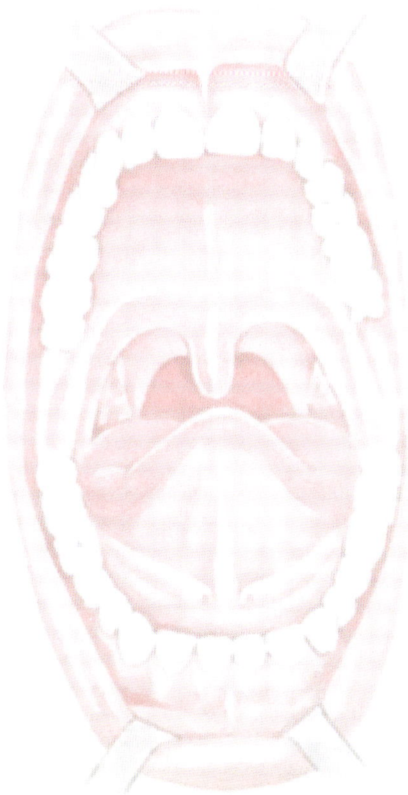

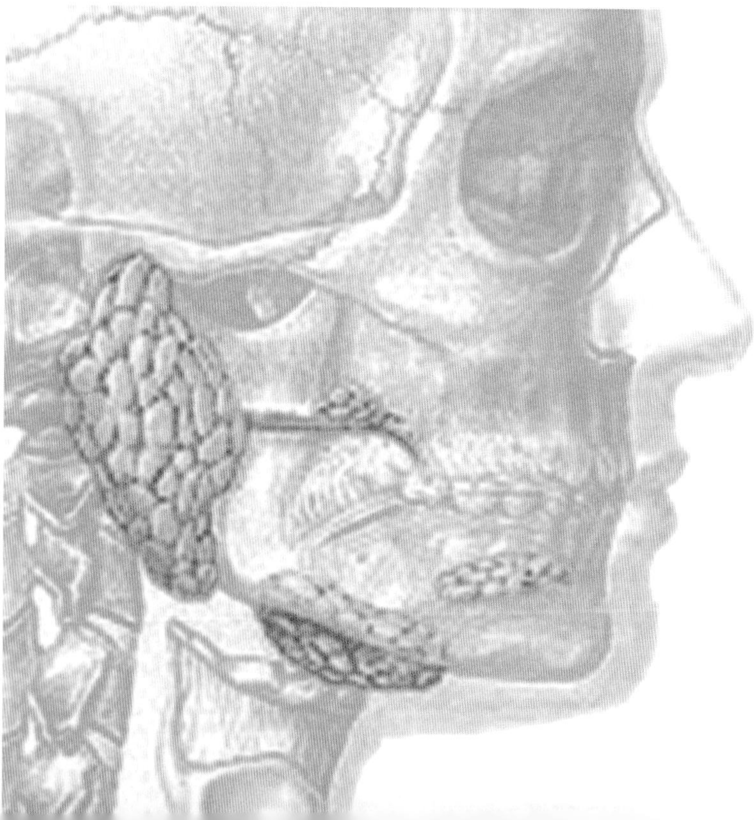

Preface

Oral physiology deals with the intricate complexities of understanding the functioning of oral and maxillofacial region. An in-depth knowledge of this field is essential for a student of dental sciences, especially at the postgraduate level, to fathom the subjectiveness of dental subjects and their followers.

Oral physiology remains the most untapped and the least understood area in dentistry and hence the requirement of this book at the postgraduate level. The demand for work of this kind remains as great as ever, keeping in view the ever evolving criteria and syllabi of postgraduate curriculum in dental sciences all over India and abroad.

Shailja Chatterjee

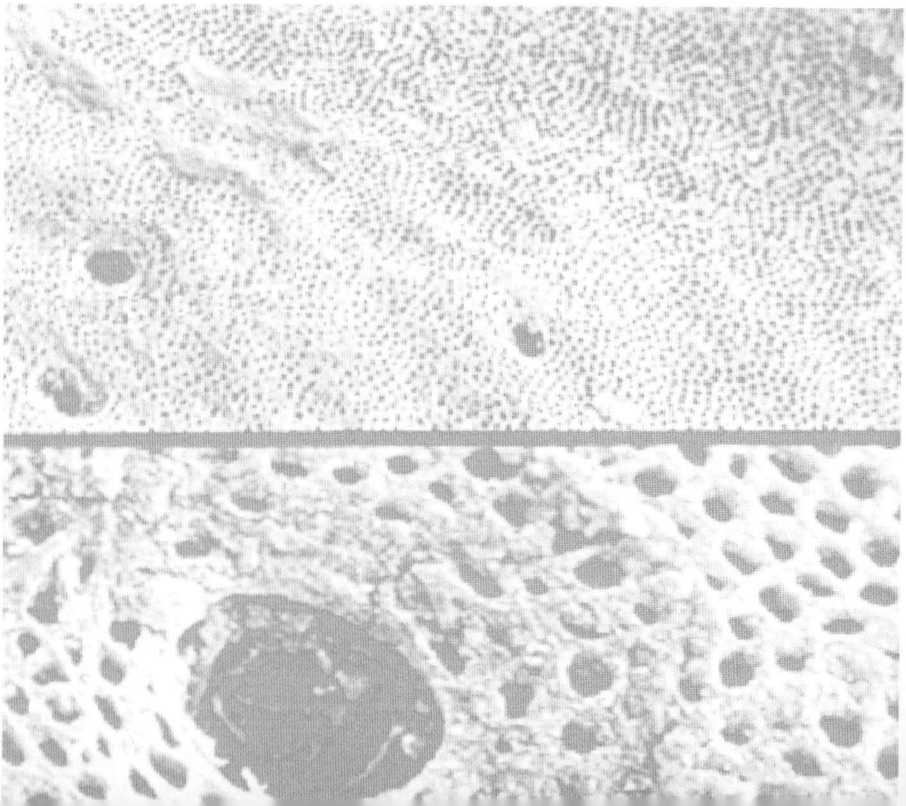

Contents

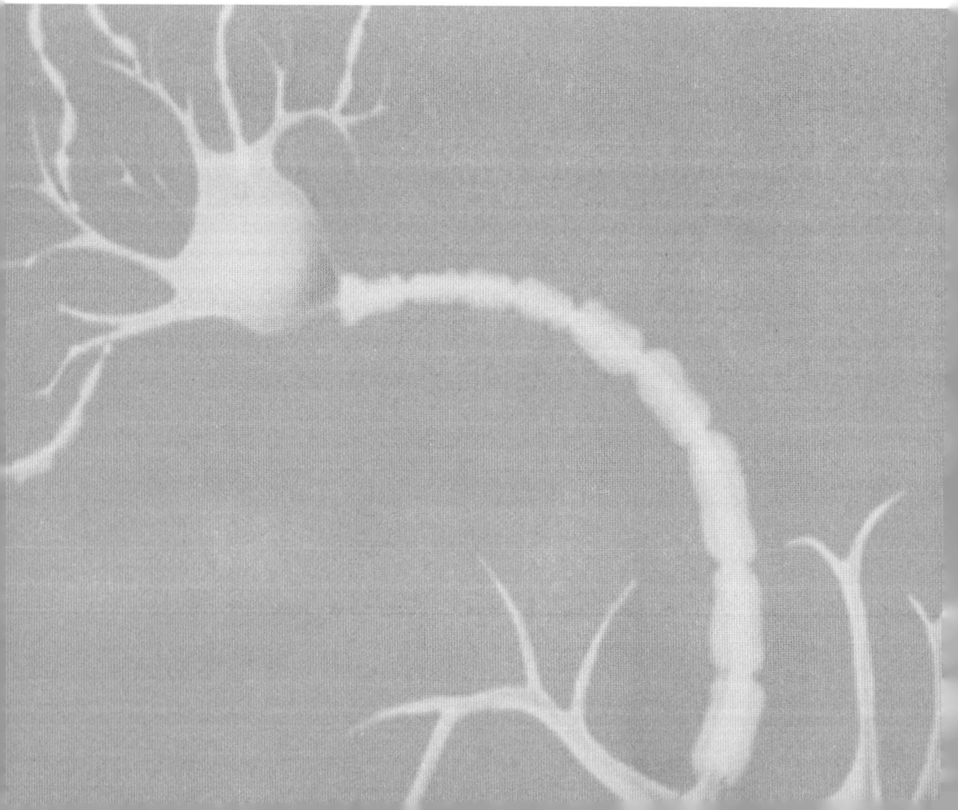

1 Saliva

Saliva is the secretory produce of all the major and minor salivary glands in the oral cavity. These glands collectively secrete up to 1 liter/day, at a flow rate which varies from 0.02 ml/min (resting saliva) to 7 ml/min or more (whole saliva).

The secretion is produced mainly by two components of the salivary gland unit—secretory acini and the ducts. In recent years, its role as an immunologically competent secretion has become important due to its constitution which comprises of immunoglobulin molecules such as secretory IgA, IgG and antibodies against viruses like HIV which can be detected with a sensitivity and specificity that are essentially identical to those of tests with serum.

The elevated concentration of these products of the immune system in saliva when compared to serum heightens its importance as an important diagnostic vis-a-vis a prognostic adjunct especially in dental caries and HIV infection.

Major Functions of Saliva

Functions	*Salivary components involved*
Protective functions	
Lubrication	Mucins, proline-like glycoproteins, water
Antimicrobial	Salivary proteins: lysozyme, lactoferrin, lactoperoxidase, mucins, cystatins, histatins, secretory IgA, proline-rich glycoproteins
Mucosal integrity	Mucins, electrolytes, water
Lavage/cleansing	Water

Buffering	Bicarbonate, phosphate ions
Remineralization	Calcium, phosphate, statherin, anionic proline-rich proteins
Food and speech-related functions	
Food preparation	Water, mucins
Digestion	Amylase, lipase, ribonuclease, protease
Taste	Water, gustin
Speech	Water, mucins

Collection of Saliva

The quantification of saliva output is referred to as "Sialometry". When measuring the flow-rate, the purpose and method of collection procedure should be explained to patient beforehand. Saliva should be collected about 1.5 to 2 hours after eating or after an overnight fast. Patient should be instructed to do nothing that might stimulate the flow of saliva prior to collection. This includes- mastication, smoking, tooth-brushing, mouthwashes, drinking, etc. The test should be conducted in a quiet area.

Analysis of Salivary Collection

To obtain mean salivary flow-rates, at least two tests should be performed, at about the same time of the day, on two different days.

If the patient's baseline has been established earlier, the values obtained can be used as a comparative indicator of the patient's salivary status. If the baseline is not known, the flow-rates have to be compared with the pertinent population standards.

As with any test, the results should be interpreted in light of the patient's history, the presence of any signs of disease and the results of other tests. Two types of measuring devices can be employed for saliva collection:

1. *Sialometer:* It is a specially constructed, re-usable device to collect both resting and stimulated saliva.
2. Any finely calibrated measuring cylinder.

Collection of Resting (unstimulated) whole Saliva

The patient is seated, head slightly down, and is asked not to swallow or move his tongue or lips during the collection period. The saliva is allowed to accumulate in mouth for 2 minutes, and he/she is then asked to spit the accumulated saliva into the receiving vessel. This procedure is performed twice more for a total of 6 minutes.

The flow-rate, expressed as ml/min = total volume of saliva (ml) divided by six minutes.

Collection of Stimulated whole Saliva

Two methods have been proposed:

1. Paraffin method
2. Citric acid method

1. *Paraffin method:* Ask the patient to hold a piece of paraffin in his mouth until it becomes soft (about 30 seconds) and then, to swallow the collected saliva. Now the patient is asked to chew the piece of wax in his usual manner of chewing for exactly 2 minutes, and then, to expectorate the accumulated saliva into the receiving vessel. The procedure is repeated twice more. The volume of saliva is read off the vessel and flow is expressed as ml/min.
2. *Citric acid method:* A 2% solution of citric acid is swabbed onto the dorsolateral surface of the tongue every 30 seconds for a period of 2 minutes. The saliva is then expectorated into the receiving vessel. As in paraffin method, the whole procedure is repeated twice more, for a total time of 6 minutes. As before, the flow is expressed as ml/min.

Collection of Saliva from Individual Major Salivary Glands

Parotid Gland

Parotid saliva is usually obtained by using several devices:

- *Carlson-Crittenden collector:* This device consists of two concentric rings of metal or plastic attached to a disc of about half an inch diameter. These tubes are inserted:
  a. Between the two rings to create a slight negative pressure.

b. Inner space which is placed over the Stensen's duct in order to lead the saliva into the receptacle placed outside the mouth.

- *Curby cup:* This is a modification of the Carlson-Crittenden collector. A third tube is included through which air bubbles can be released from the central chamber and suction of air from the outer space is effected by a rubber pipette ball fixed to a hypodermic needle inserted into the polythene tubing.

Submandibular/Sublingual Salivary Gland

For separate collection of saliva from these glands, a device designed by Schneyer (1955) is used. This device has to be specially made for each donor and consists of an acrylic appliance with three separate chambers:

- *Central chamber:* This is placed over the duct of the submandibular gland.
- *Two lateral chambers:* Cover the numerous ducts of the submandibular gland.

Disadvantages of Schneyer's apparatus:

1. Anatomical differences among individuals.
2. It cannot be used for mechanical stimuli as it projects into the ventral surface of the tongue.

Other devices employed for saliva collection:

1. Henrique and Chauncey design
2. Truelove design.

Collection of Saliva from Minor Salivary Glands

Saliva may be obtained from minor salivary glands of lower lip or palate. The minor glands are dried and isolated with a gauze or cotton rolls. After 2 minutes for resting saliva, the fluid present at the orifice of one or more of these glands is adsorbed onto filter strips (Periopaper).

The filter papers are then placed into a device (Periotron), which electronically reads the volume of fluid in each strip.

For stimulated minor gland saliva, the tongue is swabbed with a 2% citric acid solution in similar fashion. The results are expressed as ml/min.

Constituents of Saliva

Proteins

a. *Salivary protein families*

• Proline-rich	Acid, basic, glycoproteins
• Histidine-rich	Neutral, basic
• Cysteine-containing	Cystatin S, Cystatin SN
• Tyrosine-rich	Statherin
• Amylase	Glycosylated, nonglycosylated
• Mucin	
• Salivary peroxidase	

b. *Other acinar proteins*

- Lactoferrin
- Secretory component
- Zinc-binding protein: Gustin
- Parotid-aggregating glycoproteins
- Epidermal growth factor
- Antileukoprotease

c. *Serum proteins*

- Albumin
- Immunoglobulin G

d. *Ductal, stromal or unknown origin*

- Lysozyme
- Secretory IgA
- Kallikrein
- Vitamin B_{12}-binding protein
- Vitamin D-binding protein
- Fibronectin
- Nerve growth factor
- Lipase
- Ribonuclease
- Carbohydrates
- Esterases
- Amino peptidases
- Phosphatases

The total protein content of human saliva averages about 300 mg per 100 ml. The concentration in parotid is higher than in submandibular saliva and the results depend on the methods of analysis such as nitrogen estimation (Kjeldahl method), peptide links (Biuret method) or the amount of tyrosine and tryptophan.

Functional Relationship between different Salivary Molecules

Functional relationships exist between different molecules in saliva based on complexing reactions. Two types of complexing can occur:

1. *Homotypic complexing:* Between similar molecules.
2. *Heterotypic complexing:* Between different molecules.

Complexes can occur by either covalent or noncovalent interactions. For example, mucins. These molecules may form homotypic complexes or end-to-end oligomers, with themselves via interchain disulfide bonds. For example, mucin oligomer formation is required for this molecule to exert its lubrication and viscoelastic properties. Mucins that coat various oral tissue surfaces can also form heterotypic complexes with other salivary molecules, including sIgA, lysosomes and cystatins.

These complexes are mediated primarily by noncovalent ionic forces and function to concentrate these antimicrobials at saliva-tissue interface.

GLYCOPROTEINS

Proline, Glycine and Glutamic Acid-rich Glycoproteins

About 80% of amino acids secreted in saliva are made of proline, glycine and glutamic acid. The carbohydrate content comprises of approximately equal proportions of N-acetyl glucosamine, mannose, galactose and fucose with small amounts of sialate.

When rapidly secreted, the protein core is present without its carbohydrate chains; presumably, it is secreted before carbohydrate groups get attached.

Blood Group-active Glycoproteins

a. *Salivary mucins:* Human saliva contains two genetically distinct mucin subtypes; designated MG1 and MG2 originating from MUC5B and MUC7 gene, respectively.

- MG1 (MUC5B): This glycoprotein displays blood group activity. It exists in at least 3 different glycoforms, differing in sialic acid and sulfate content depending on glandular source. Different MUC5B glycoforms can be isolated with one glandular secretion.

  MUC5B functionally and structurally belongs to the classic mucins, which are the main constituents of slime layers covering mucous epithelia throughout the body. These secretory mucins, although encompassing a genetically heterogenous family, have a comparable architecture. They are composed of disulphide linked monomers that are heavily glycosylated peptide domains ('naked' domains). Because of their carbohydrate content (>80%), their larger dimensions (>1µm), and their extended thread-like structure, the classical secretory mucins already at low concentrations form hydrophilic viscoelastic gels. These gels function as barriers protecting the underlying epithelium against mechanical damage and preventing direct entrance of noxious agents into the epithelium.

  In the oral cavity, MUC5B is present in the protein fibers (pellicles) covering the enamel and epithelial surfaces, thereby, protecting them against acidic attacks.

- MG2 (MUC7): MUG2 is found to exist in two glycoforms, MG2a and MG2b, respectively.

  In contrast to MUC5B, the carbohydrate side-chains of MUC7 are predominantly, sialyted di- and trisaccharides. Furthermore, MUC7 lacks blood group active carbohydrates of the ABO system, a feature that is considered a characteristic feature of mucins.

  MUC7 and the salivary agglutinins are among the major bacteria-agglutinating factors in saliva. For example, *Streptococcus sanguis, S.mitis, S.gordonii, Actinobacillus actinomycetemcomitans, Pseudomonas aeruginosa* and *Escherichia coli.*

Agglutinins

Salivary agglutinin is a highly glycosylated protein, with a molecular mass of approximately 340 kDa, that carries blood group active antigens. Both MUC7 and salivary agglutinin are expressed in the serous cells of submandibular, sublingual and lingual glands. However, agglutinin in contrast to MUC7, is also synthesized in serous parotid gland.

Agglutinins are synthesized only in ductal cells in parotids, whereas in the submandibular gland agglutinin was detected in both serous acinar and demilune cells capping the mucous acini.

Agglutinins like MUC7 bind to a wide variety of microorganisms including *S. mutans, S. salivarius* and *S. sanguis*.

Cystatins (cysteine proteinase inhibitors)

These proteins have been classified as members of family 2 cystatins. In saliva, at least nine different cystatin isoforms are secreted, including:

a. Neutral cystatin SN
b. Three moderately anionic isoforms of cystatin SA
c. 3 or 4 isoforms of the more anionic cystatin S
d. Cystatin C, cationic cystatin
e. Cystatin D.

Cystatins have been suggested to play a role in controlling proteolytic activity, either from the host (released during inflammatory process) or from microorganisms.

Cystatin C, although a minor constituent of the total population of oral cystatins, contributes most to the cysteine proteinase inhibitory activity of saliva.

Von Ebner Glands Protein

This is a salivary protein secreted by von Ebner glands located around the circumvallate and foliate papillae of the tongue. It is also known as *tear-specific prealbumin*. This protein has numerous functions:

a. Perception of bitter taste by binding lipophilic bitter compounds and transporting them to taste buds.

b. It acts as an inhibitor of cysteine proteinase.
c. It can act as an oxidative-stress induced scavenger of peroxidation products.
d. It has an endonuclease activity acting on viral cells.

SLPI (secretory leukocyte proteinase inhibitor)

This is an inhibitor of serine proteinase (serpin), including neutrophil elastase, chymotrypsin and Cathepsin G.

Amylase

Amylase (46–60kDa) is an abundant salivary component. This enzyme catalyzes hydrolysis of α(1,4)-glycosidic binding between glucose residues of polysaccharides (e.g. starch, glycogen, and dextrins). Human amylase exists in 2 forms:

a. Pancreatic
b. Salivary glands

These two forms have 97% amino acid homology. Amylase displays growth-inhibiting activity against *N. gonnorhoea*. However, in *S. gordonii*, amylase allows the microbe to utilize starch as a carbohydrate source.

Antimicrobial Peptides (histatins and defensins)

In human saliva, at least 12 histatin-like peptides have been identified, the majority of which are degradation fragments of two parent molecules, Histatin 1 and 3. Of all histatins, histatin 1, 3 and 5 (derived from histatin 3) are most abundant in parotid saliva. Histatin 5 has numerous properties:

a. Fungicidal
b. Bactericidal
c. Pellicle formation
d. Neutralization of potentially harmful pathogens.

Acinar Proteins

a. *Lactoferrin:* The presence of lactoferrin in secretions such as saliva, tears and milk is usually linked with its iron-binding properties. This is responsible for the bacteriostatic effect of saliva. One of the target microorganism of lactoferrin is the periopathogenic bacterium, *A. actinomycetemcomitans*. It has been reported that in periodontitis patients carrying *A. actinomycetemcomitans*, a negative correlation exists between the number of subgingival *A. actinomycetemcomitans* and the lactoferrin concentration in saliva. In addition, it inhibits the growth of *Helicobacter pylori* in an *in vitro* culture system and *H. felis* in an *in vivo* mouse model.

Antimicrobial domains are released during lactoferrin digestion in gastrointestinal tract, therefore, playing a protective role.

It is now proven that lactoferrin is a multifunctional protein having bacteriostatic, bactericidal, fungicidal, antiviral, anti-inflammatory and immunomodulatory properties.

b. *Extra-parotid glycoprotein (EP-GP):* EP-GP is another example of a protein that originally has been implicated in the formation of dental pellicle, because of its high affinity for hydroxyapatite.

   It has a ubiquitous presence in mucosal secretions like sweat, semen and tears. This protein binds to microorganisms as well as to the CD4 receptors on monocytes.

c. *Secretory immunoglobulin (sIgA):* sIgA is a member of the adaptive immune response. It is the predominant immunoglobulin of the mucosal immune system. In addition, the sIgA production (± 66 mg/kg/day) is greater than that of the other isotypes of immunoglobulins. This high production is necessary to cover the epithelial surfaces of the body.

   This immunoglobulin is synthesized by B-lymphocytes and is composed of 2 four-chain units of IgA, one secretory component and one joining (J) chain. Local stimulation as well as common mucosal immune response are responsible for its production. However, no correlation has been found between sIgA deficiency and periodontal disease probably due to compensation by elevated IgG and IgM levels.

d. *Zinc-α2-glycoprotein:* This consists of a single polypeptide chain with 18% carbohydrate. It precipitates zinc ions and constitutes a minor component in saliva.

Other Salivary Proteins

a. *Kallikrein:* Kallikreins are a group of serine proteases that are found in glandular cells, neutrophils, and biological fluids. The function of this enzyme is the cleavage of kininogen into kinin. Glandular (tissue) kallikrein is found in a variety of tissues and biological fluids, including saliva. In saliva, this protein has numerous functions:
   - Hydrolytic activity on proline-rich proteins.
   - Regulation of blood flow in salivary glands.
   - Processing of polypeptide hormones like Epidermal Growth Factor.
   - Ion transport in epithelial cells.
   - Neutrophil chemotaxis: High amounts of this protein have been noted in subjects with tumors as compared to control.

b. *Lysozyme:* Also known as Muramidase, was first recognized by Fleming (1920) for its bactericidal properties. It belongs to the innate immune response arm and acts by cleaving β(1,4)-glycosidic bonds between muramic acid and N-acetylglucosamine residues in the peptidoglycans of the bacterial cell wall. The majority of bacterial species are not directly lysed upon exposure to lysozyme, but their cell walls become weakened to such an extent that subsequent addition of anions or detergents results in immediate lysis.

   Studies have shown that the binding of host-inactivated lysozyme to bacterial cells is sufficient to induce killing and lysis.

c. *Lactoperoxidases:* The peroxidase activity of saliva is derived from 2 sources:
   - Human salivary lactoperoxidase: It is synthesized and secreted by salivary glands.
   - Myeloperoxidase: It is found in PMNLs, which migrate into the oral cavity through gingival crevices. The contribution of myeloperoxidase to the total salivary peroxidases varies between 30 to 75% depending upon oral health of the subjects. Salivary peroxidases catalyze the formation of bactericidal compounds such as hypothiocyanate.

d. *Chitinase:* Chitinase catalyzes the hydrolytic cleavage of chitin which is a cell wall component of yeasts. Therefore, it has a protective role against fungal colonization of oral epithelium. Studies have shown significant levels in periodontitis patients as compared to normal subjects. Thereby suggesting that its expression is regulated by inflammatory mediators.

Formation and Secretion of Saliva

The formation of saliva occurs in two stages:

1. *First stage:* Cells of the secretory end pieces and the intercalated ducts produce isotonic saliva or primary saliva.
2. *Second stage:* The primary saliva is modified as it passes through striated and excretory ducts, mainly by resorption and secretion of electrolytes. The final saliva that is secreted in oral cavity is hypotonic.

Protein Secretion

Protein secretion occurs by exocytosis, i.e., fusion of secretory granules with luminal surface to release their contents into the lumen. The binding of sympathetic neurotransmitter norepinephrin (NE) to β-adrenergic receptors (β) on the basolateral membrane activates adenylyl cyclase (AC), which catalyzes the formation of cAMP from ATP. cAMP activates protein kinase A (PKA), which phosphorylates other proteins in a cascade leading to exocytosis.

Fluid and Electrolyte Secretion

Fluid and electrolyte secretion is stimulated mainly by the binding of the parasympathetic transmitter, acetylcholine (ACh) to muscarinic cholinergic receptors, and by norepinephrin binding to α-receptors. These receptors activate phospholipase C (PLC), which converts phospatidylinositol biphosphate (PIP_2) to inositol triphosphate (IP_3) and diacylglycerol (DAG). IP_3 causes the release of calcium ions from intracellular stores, e.g. endoplasmic reticulum.

The increased calcium concentration opens chloride channels in the luminal membrane and potassium channels in the basolateral membrane, and activates the basolateral $Na^+/K^+/2Cl^-$ cotransporter. The increased luminal Cl^- is balanced by the movement of the basolateral $Na^+/K^+/2Cl^-$ cotransporter and Na^+/K^+-ATPase serve to maintain the intracellular electrolyte and osmotic balances.

Calcium also stimulates exocytosis but to a lesser degree than cAMP, and it modulates the activity of protein kinase A and PKC. Protein kinase C, in turn, modulates exocytosis and intracellular calcium concentrations.

Diagnostic uses of Saliva

Oncology

a. *p53:* p53 is a tumor suppressor gene expressed during genotoxic damage. Inactivation of this gene through mutations and deletions results in development of cancers. The accumulation of inactive p53 results in production of

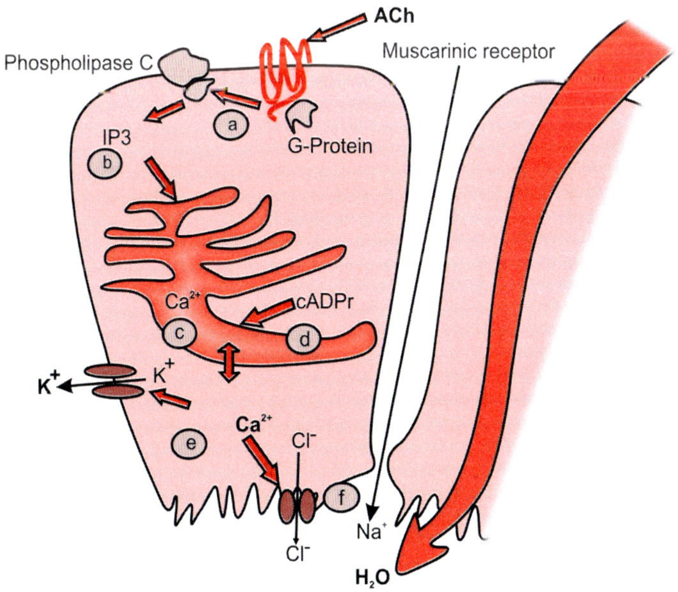

Fig. 1.1: Diagrammatic representation of fluid and electrolyte movements within a salivary ductal cell in response to acetylcholine enzyme

antibodies against this protein which are detectable in sera of patients.

It is detectable in saliva of patients diagnosed with oral squamous cell carcinoma, and can thus assist in early detection and screening of oral cancer.

b. *Defensins:* An elevated level of salivary defensin-1 is an indicator of oral squamous cell carcinoma.

c. *C-erb-B2 and Cancer Antigen 15-3 (CA15-3):* These tumor markers have been detected in saliva of patients with breast cancer.

d. *CA125:* CA125 is a tumor marker for epithelial ovarian carcinoma. Elevated salivary levels of CA125 have been detected in ovarian carcinoma patients.

Hereditary Diseases

Cystic fibrosis is a genetically transmitted disease and is considered a generalized exocrinopathy. The gene defect causing CF is present on chromosome 7 and codes for a transmembrane-regulating protein called *cystic fibrosis transmembrane conductance regulator.*

Saliva of CF patients contains increased calcium levels. Elevated levels of calcium and phosphorus in submandibular saliva results in calcium-protein aggregation, which causes increased turbidity of saliva. This may explain a higher occurrence of calculus in cystic fibrosis patients as compared to controls (normal individuals).

The submandibular saliva in CF patients has also been found to contain elevated lipid levels. For example, neutral lipids; phospholipids, and glycolipids.

Decreased protease activity in saliva from CF patients has been observed as compared to healthy controls. An Epidermal Growth actor (EGF) has been found in saliva of CF patients. However, detection of carriers (heterozygotes) for CF patients is not possible through salivary analysis and is therefore, a limitation in use of saliva as a diagnostic tool in such subjects.

Autoimmune Diseases

Sjögren's syndrome: Sialochemistry is an important tool in the diagnosis of Sjögren's syndrome. Findings include: Increased levels of sodium and chloride, IgA, IgG, lactoferrin, α2-microglobulin and cystatin S/C and decreased levels of phosphates.

Infectious Diseases

a. *H. pylori* infection: *H. pylori* infection is associated with peptic ulcer and chronic gastritis. An ELISA test for detection of IgG antibody in serum produced 97% sensitivity and 94% specificity in detection of this disease. This indicates an oral route of transmission of *H. pylori*.

b. *Lyme disease:* This is caused by spirochaete, *Borrelia burgdorferi* and is transmitted to humans by ticks. The detection of anti-tick antibody in saliva has potential as a biological marker for screening of individuals at risk of Lyme disease.

HIV

Studies have demonstrated an equal efficacy of saliva to serum in diagnosis and screening of HIV. Salivary IgA levels have been found to decline as infected patients become symptomatic. The advantage of saliva as a diagnostic and prognostic tool in HIV diagnosis is the non-invasive nature of collection, which eliminates the risk of infection in the health care workers as viral transmission via saliva does not take place.

References

1. Schramm W, Angulo GA, Torres PC, Cassler AB. A Simple Saliva-Based Test for Detecting Antibodies to Human Immunodeficiency Virus. Clin Diagn Lab Immunol; 1999; July:577–80.
2. Emmons W. Accuracy of oral specimen testing for human immunodeficiency virus. Am. J. Med. 1997;102 (Suppl. 4A):15–20.
3. Hodinka, RL, T Nagashunmugan, D. Malamud. Detection of human immunodeficiency virus antibodies in oral fluids. Clin. Diagn. Lab. Immunol. 1998;5:419–26.
4. Clark GW and Levine L. Inorganic constituents of human saliva (II), Amer. J. Physiol. 1927;81,264–70.
5. Eisenbrandt LL. Studies on the pH of saliva. J of Dent Res. 1943;22:147.

2 Mineralization

INTRODUCTION

Calcification: Refers to the deposition of calcium phosphate in bone and teeth, although most of the hypotheses suggest to have involved an active participation of phosphate more than calcium.

Mineralization: It is a more satisfactory term than calcification and refers to deposition of any mineral salt.

Types of Mechanisms

1. Booster mechanism
2. Seeding theory

Booster mechanism: It involves enzymatic activity which by further increase would cause a rise in calcium or phosphorus concentration, which by law of mass action, leads to precipitation.

Seeding theory: The presence of a seeding or 'nucleating' substance which, because its shape resembles that of apatite, acts as a mould or template upon which the crystals are laid down (this seeding process is known as 'epitaxy') following which crystallization proceeds automatically.

THEORIES OF MINERALIZATION

Robison's Alkaline Phosphatase Theory

This theory is no longer held in its original form. The discovery of enzyme 'Alkaline Phosphatase' in mineralizing tissues suggested that this enzyme released inorganic phosphate from organic phosphates (e.g. hexose phosphate), thereby, raising the concentration of phosphate ions locally. These raised phosphate ions react with calcium ions in the tissue fluid, leading to the precipitation of insoluble calcium phosphate.

$$\text{Calcium phosphate} \xrightarrow{\text{Alkaline phosphatase}} \text{Calcium + Phosphate ions}$$

This precipitation occurs in following stages:

$Ca^{2+} + HPO_4^{2-} \rightarrow$ amorphous calcium phosphate $\rightarrow$ Apatite

It is not certain whether releasing phosphate into a medium supersaturated with calcium phosphate leads to precipitation, but it does increase the degree of supersaturation.

Points Favoring Theory

When slices of cartilage, dissected from bones of young rachitic rats, are incubated with solution containing calcium ions and organic phosphates (split by phosphatase), the calcium phosphate is laid down in a way similar to histologic normal calcification. This technique is referred to as **calcification *in vitro***.

Drawbacks

1. The results obtained in the above experiment are in rachitic tissues but not applied to normal bone.
2. Alkaline phosphatase is found in tissues which do not calcify.
3. Certain enzyme inhibitors which do not affect phosphatase, inhibit calcification *in vitro*.
4. *in vitro* calcification occurs in solutions containing calcium ions and inorganic phosphate (i.e. in absence of organic phosphates).

Cartier's Adenosine Triphosphate Theory

Cartier studied the calcification of bone slices from lamb embryos and obtained very different results from Robison's study on rat's rachitic cartilage. This difference in both the studies can be attributed to two reasons:

a. Species difference.

b. Difference in technique.

ATP is extremely powerful in inducing mineralization due to splitting into pyrophosphate (PP_i) and subsequently into inorganic phosphate (P_i).

$$ATP \xrightarrow{\text{Pyrophosphatase}} PP_i \xrightarrow{\text{Pyrophosphatase}} P_i$$

Even synthetic apatite and reconstituted collagen fibers may act as a catalyst with an action similar to that of alkaline phosphatase.

$$ATP \xrightarrow{\text{Apatite/Collagen}} P_i$$

Seeding Theory

Collagen fibers reconstituted from collagen solution, if placed in a medium supersaturated with calcium and phosphate ions, appear to act as seeds for apatite crystals to form on fibers. Proteins such as gelatin and fibrin, do not induce crystal formation.

Nature of Seeding Process

There are two ways in which a molecule induces crystallization:

Different regions of the molecule might have a distribution of electric charges.

This distribution of charges or spatial configuration of seeds may encourage calcium and phosphate ions to combine at positions similar to those occupied in colloidal calcium phosphate or in some salts, such as $CaHPO_4$, which may precipitate first and then convert to apatite.

Nature of Seed

A wide variety of substances can act as a seed *in vitro* for hydroxyapatite deposition and it is quite probable that more than one naturally occurring substance is active *in vitro.*

The following substances have been considered as possible seeding substances in bone:

1. *Collagen:* Glimcher observed that only fibers showing 640Å banding are mineralized *in vitro*. If these fibers are swollen

by exposure to acid or alkali, or shrunken by heat (i.e., their orderly structure is destroyed), they lose their power to act as seed.

Electron micrographs show that when crystals have grown large enough to be detected, they tend to lie 640Å apart, i.e. they show a definite relationship to the bands, so that the early crystal, at least, seems to be related to some structure having a periodicity similar to collagen.

Calculation of the volume of collagen and mineral matter in the fully-mineralized tissues strongly suggests that some of the mineral must be within the collagen fibers since the spaces between the fibers are too small to accommodate the amount of mineral present. The seeding of apatite inside the fibers has also been seen in electron micrographs and it has been suggested that seeding might occur in the **holes** in the collagen fibers.

The collagen does not nucleate if its carboxylic ends are blocked by converting them into amides, presumably calcium binds to the carboxylic groups. Therefore, the presence of carboxylic groups is required to induce seeding.

Collagen from mineralizing tissues differs from that of non-mineralizing tissues by the spaces between the collagen molecules in bone and dentin by an average of 6Å. But since reconstituted fibers from both mineralizing and non-mineralizing tissues are found to mineralize *in vitro*, it is supposed that in course of reconstitution, these differences disappear. A suggested opinion is that non-mineralizing tissues contain an inhibitor of mineralization. The evidence for this theory is as follows:

a. If collagen is placed in solutions varying in calcium and phosphate concentration, it is possible to find the minimum product (Ca concentration) × (P_i concentration) at which mineralization occurs. If plasma is included in medium, the (Ca concentration) × (P_i concentration) product at which mineralization occurred arose, suggesting the presence of an inhibitor in plasma.

   Inhibition can be induced by ATP, pyrophosphate and tripolyphosphate suggesting the presence of naturally occurring inhibitors of mineralization. It has been demonstrated that plasma that has been previously incubated with alkaline phosphatase shows no inhibitory effect. However, this view is contraindicated by the absence of mineralization from many tissues (e.g. kidney and intestine) which contains both alkaline phosphatase and collagen.

b. Although reconstituted collagen with 640Å band readily mineralizes in solutions saturated with calcium and phosphate ions, studies on crude collagen from skin have been shown to either not mineralize at all or do so less readily. This can be attributed to certain changes in collagen structure due to removal of certain substances from collagen during dissolution and reconstitution.

2. *Chondroitin sulfate:* Chondroitin sulfate is the most acidic substance in calcifying tissues and it has been speculated that it may act as a seed *in vivo*. This idea has been supported by experiments in which substances capable of combining strongly with chondroitin sulfate were found to inhibit calcification *in vitro*.

   Drawbacks:

   a. Collagen fibers reconstituted from pure solutions containing no chondroitin sulfate act as seeds in calcifying solution.

   b. Hyaline cartilage is one of the chondroitin sulfate-rich tissues but it does not necessarily calcify, whereas in bone the concentration is much lower.

3. *Lipid substance associated with seed:* A substance which stains as a lipid with Sudan black has been detected in areas of active mineralization of bone and teeth. It has also been reported in areas of resorption in bone and dentin of resorbing deciduous roots. It exists in tissues in a form which does not stain unless treated with pyridine or alcohol which 'unmasks' it by removing a substance which protects it. Analysis of lipids in mineralizing tissues show them to be a complicated mixture of triglycerides, free fatty acids, and various phospholipids, about half of which contains serine or inositol.

When lipids from a variety of tissues are added to metastable solutions of calcium phosphate, a precipitate forms consisting largely of apatite, but consisting of 1.9% lipids.

This lipid cannot be extracted from the precipitate unless the apatite is dissolved first, suggesting some form of binding. If different lipids are added separately to mineralizing solutions, only the phospholipids have been found to precipitate apatite.

4. *Phosphoproteins:* Phosphoproteins are a group of conjugated proteins, in which a phosphate group is attached to serine. These have been proposed to act as seeds, particularly in dentin. It has been suggested that serine group of collagen or of a specific protein in the mineralizing tissues becomes phosphorylated by the action of enzyme, *protein phosphokinase*, which transfers a phosphate group from ATP to the protein. Phosphoproteins are known to be present in the mineralizing tissues and might be expected to attract calcium and thus become nucleating centres.

   Drawbacks:

   a. There is little evidence for this hypotheses.
   b. Phosphoproteins are found in milk and egg yolk where mineralization does not occur.

Matrix Vesicle Theory

Electron micrographs of developing cartilage show groups of round or ovoid, osmophillic vesicles between 500–2500Å in diameter near each cell. In cartilage with well advanced mineralization, these vesicles contain crystals identified by X-ray diffraction as apatite. The clusters of crystals grow and coalesce until the whole matrix is mineralized. If the section is demineralized by EDTA or acids and treated with lead citrate or other fixatives, the crystals disappear but 'ghosts' of organic matter remain–evidently the apatite crystals are closely associated with organic matter. There are two types of vesicles:

1. Type I
2. Type II.

Type I: Vesicles are round or oval in shape, resembling lysosomes. They contain acid phosphatase and aryl sulfatase which breakdown the proteoglycans and glycosaminoglycans (GAGs) whose concentrations are known to fall as mineralization occurs.

Type II: Vesicles are irregular in shape and bound by a trimellar membrane, sometimes containing ribosomes and have an internal structure resembling cytoplasm. They contain alkaline phosphatase and ATPase, which are enzymes characteristic of cartilage cells and lipids, chiefly *phosphatidylserine*, a substance previously shown in lipids of the 'calcifying' front. This substance has a strong affinity for calcium, especially in presence of phosphate and it has been speculated that it is important in concentrating calcium ions, thus acting as a 'seed'.

Alkaline phosphatase (also known as "tissue non-specific alkaline phosphatase") was first identified in 1923 by Robison, who was the first to suggest its activity in calcium phosphate mineral deposition.

It seems that Type II vesicles may promote mineralization in several ways by involving all the previous hypotheses proposed. The alkaline phosphatase has pyrophosphatase activity. It converts the inhibitor 'pyrophosphate' (PP_i) into orthophosphate, thus removing its inhibitory power and simultaneously converting it into a booster by increasing the concentration of orthophosphate. The lipid may attract calcium ions, this action being favored by the orthophosphate which, in turn, will be available to convert the calcium into calcium phosphate.

The presence of ATPase suggests that the reactions proposed by Cartier may occur in the vesicles. Alternatively, ATPase may be concerned with an energy-requiring calcium transport system as in the cells of the intestine.

One proposed hypotheses regarding mineralization suggests that amorphous calcium phosphate is precipitated in the vesicles which, being more soluble than hydroxyapatite crystals, dissolves by unknown mechanisms in the tissue fluid surrounding the cells of the mineralizing tissue. The calcium and phosphate ions then diffuse into the collagen fibers because, in the mineralizing tissues, the spaces between the fibers are large enough to permit these ions to enter, where they form a hydroxyapatite by seeding pattern. In other words, the vesicles carry out a concentrating process which provides the collagen with sufficient ions to form hydroxyapatite crystals.

MECHANISM OF MATRIX VESICLE MINERALIZATION

It would appear that mineralization, as initiated by matrix vesicles, is essentially a biphasic phenomenon.

Phase 1 is concerned with the formation of the first crystals of mineral within matrix vesicles. This phase probably begins with the absorption of Ca^{2+} into the matrix vesicles membranes and then into the matrix vesicle sap, due to a local enrichment of Ca-binding phospholipids and proteins in matrix vesicles plus the inward Ca^{2+} transporting activity of Annexin V. Inward Ca^{2+} transport would be accompanied by PO_4^{3-} accumulation within the matrix vesicle, as augmented by the phosphate concentrating activities of the Na-PO_4 transporter plus the enzymatic activity of phospho1, which appears to play an early role in phosphate concentration by matrix vesicles .

Alkaline phosphatase activity also may function in the early accumulation of phosphate within matrix vesicles, but seems to be more important in providing an enrichment of phosphate at the perimeter of matrix vesicles during early **Phase 2** mineral propagation. In all likelihood, Ca^{2+} and PO_4^{3-} accumulation within matrix vesicles overlaps to some degree. When sufficient Ca^{2+} and PO_4^{3-} have accumulated within the matrix vesicles, calcium phosphate mineral will begin to precipitate. The first calcium phosphate deposited is a non-crystalline form, i.e. amorphous calcium phosphate (ACP). ACP is thought to convert to octacalcium phosphate, whose crystals are then transformed into the highly insoluble hydroxyapatite. Hydroxyapatite crystals must penetrate the matrix vesicle membrane and be exposed to the extracellular fluid in order to initiate phase 2. Matrix vesicle membrane breakdown may be assisted by the hydrolytic action of phospholipases and proteases that have been identified in matrix vesicles.

Phase 1 of mineral initiation thus reflects a cascade of multiple molecular interactions that occur within matrix vesicles because of their unique molecular composition and three-dimensional membrane structure.

Phase 2 begins with crystal penetration of the matrix vesicle membrane, thus exposing preformed mineral crystals to the extracellular fluid. The rate of mineral crystal proliferation is governed by extravesicular fluid conditions such as the levels of ionic calcium and phosphate ions in the extracellular fluid at the site of mineral initiation, the pH of the extracellular fluid, and the presence of molecules in the extracellular fluid that can control the rate of mineral crystal propagation.

Included in this group of extravesicular mineralization-regulating molecules are:

1. Collagen types I and II, both of which can promote mineral proliferation.
2. Calcium-binding matrix proteins including bone sialoprotein, which have the ability to promote mineralization while osteonectin and osteocalcin may retard mineralization.
3. Acidic Calcium-binding proteoglycans of the extracellular matrix which bind and sequester ionic Ca^{2+}, thus inhibiting mineral propagation into the growth plate cartilage matrix.
4. The local concentration of extravesicular phosphoester substrates for matrix vesicle phosphatases, including ATP, AMP and PPi.

All three of these phosphoesters are hydrolyzed to yield inorganic phosphate for incorporation into propagating mineral by the enzymatic activity of ALP, which is attached to the outer surfaces of the matrix vesicle membrane. An over-abundance of extracellular PPi would tend to inhibit mineral propagation, while physiologic levels of PPi, in the micromolar range, would tend to promote mineralization.

Phase 2 mineral propagation continues with the accumulation of new self-nucleated crystals of hydroxyapatite to form spherical clusters at the surfaces of matrix vesicles.

This spherical pattern of early mineral accumulation around matrix vesicles in growth plates is also seen in newly formed bone, in dentin, and in calcifying tendons.

After a short period, the proliferating extra-vesicular crystals come into contact with collagen fibrils of the surrounding matrix. At this point collagen begins to play a major role in nucleating and orienting newly formed apatite crystals. In the growth plate, the transfer of mineral-nucleating activity from matrix vesicles to collagen is facilitated by matrix proteins, which provide a molecular bridge between matrix vesicles and collagen type II fibrils. These bridging proteins include proteoglycan link protein and proteoglycans hydroxyapatite binding region. Crystals that are generated within and at the surfaces of collagen fibrils form in coalignment with the typical 64 nanometer axial periodicity of the collagen fibrils. Thus, there is persuasive experimental evidence indicating that matrix vesicles and type I or II collagen fibrils work synergistically to achieve the full mineralization of cartilage and bone matrix.

NEW EVIDENCE OF NON-MINERALIZING FUNCTIONS OF MATRIX VESICLES

Bone Morphogenetic Proteins (BMP)

BMPs have recently been identified in matrix vesicles in significant quantities by Western blots, using proteins from cartilage growth plate. Although the finding of BMPs in growth plate matrix vesicles is preliminary and needs to be confirmed, it has important implications because it suggests that matrix vesicles of the growth plate may function as carriers of important morphogenetic information delivered to the subjacent metaphysis where new bone is forming. This finding is reminiscent of the suggestion advanced several years ago by Slavkin, *et al* (1972), who proposed that matrix vesicles may function as carriers of morphogenetic signals during tooth development.

Thus, in the case of the growth plate, matrix vesicles also may function as carriers of morphogenetic signals, such as BMPs, that are involved in signaling uncommitted osteoprogenitor cells subjacent to the growth plate to undergo osseous differentiation. The BMPs carried by matrix vesicles to the hypertrophic matrix at the base of the growth plate would be released from the matrix during the vascularization and cartilage matrix resorption that occurs actively at this level. BMPs in matrix vesicles may in fact stimulate resorption of the growth plate by activating osteoclasts. It has recently been shown that osteoclasts are stimulated by BMP–2 and –4, via BMP receptors on osteoclasts. BMP receptors are also required for osteoclastogenesis.

Matrix Metalloproteinases (MMPs) and Peptidases

MMPs and peptidases, known to be present in matrix vesicles may not only promote mineralization but also regulate bone morphogenesis. Regarding mineralization, it was shown earlier that matrix vesicles are enriched in neutral peptidases and metalloproteinases. These proteinases have the ability to digest proteoglycans of growth plate cartilage matrix. Studies by Dziewaitkowski and Majznerski (1985) showed quite clearly that aggregates of acidic proteoglycans inhibit calcification during endochondral ossification, more than do proteoglycan monomers. Furthermore, it is known that proteoglycans of the growth plate become less aggregated as they approach the calcifying zone of the growth plate. Disaggregation and digestion of proteoglycans in the calcifying zone of growth plates is likely due to the release of proteases both from matrix vesicles and from apoptotic chondrocytes, thus promoting phase 2 mineralization. More recently, it has been shown that matrix vesicles isolated from chick growth plate contain active MMPs, and are particularly enriched in MMP–2, –9 and –13. MMP–2 and 9 are particularly enriched in tumor cells generated vesicles.

Matrix metalloproteinases –2 and –9 are gelatinases, while MMP–13 is a collagenase that is concentrated in the hypertrophic chondrocytes. A null mutation of MMP-9 inhibits apoptosis of hypertrophic chondrocytes, thus causing a five-fold enlargement of the hypertrophic zone of the mouse growth plate, plus a failure of vascular invasion from the metaphysis.

It is hypothesized that MMP–9 deficiency impedes release and activation of MMP–13 from hypertrophic chondrocytes. MMP–13, which is attached to the surfaces of matrix vesicle membranes plus MMP–9 work synergistically to facilitate the release and dispersion of vascular endothelial growth factor (VEGF) from terminal, apoptotic chondrocytes. VEGF is an angiogenic factor, highly expressed in hypertrophic chondrocytes, that promotes vascular in-growth as well as osteoclast recruitment to the base of the growth plate, where active resorption of cartilage matrix precedes the in-growth of new bone. MMP–13 is also capable of activating transforming growth factor (TGF)-beta, which regulates chondrocyte proliferation and differentiation in the growth plate. Thus, MMPs that are concentrated in matrix vesicles, especially MMP–9 and –13, working together, appear to have an important role in promoting chondrocyte growth and differentiation, plus vascular invasion, and cartilage matrix resorption, during cartilage replacement by in-growing bone, at the base of the growth plate.

MINERALIZATION OF ENAMEL

Enamel Proteins

The organic matrix of enamel is made from noncollagenous protein and contains several enamel proteins and enzymes. Of the enamel proteins, 90% are a heterogenous group of low molecular weight proteins known as **amelogenins**. The remaining 10% consists of nonamelogenins such as enamelin and ameloblastin.

Amelogenin

Amelogenins are hydrophobic proteins rich in proline, histidine and glutamine, showing little post-translational modifications and molecular weights ranging between 5 and 45 kDa. Their heterogeneity is brought about in three ways:

1. The genes responsible for transcribing amelogenin are found on X and Y-chromosomes, and because these two genes are not 100% homologous, a sexual heterogeneity exists. The functional significance of this sexual dimorphism is not known.
2. The amelogenin gene contains at least seven exons, which can be spliced in numerous ways to produce mRNAs. Spliced

mRNA fragments may include all the seven exons or lack some of them. The functional significance of alternately spliced forms of amelogenin is not known.

3. Amelogenins undergo short-term (minor) and long-term (extensive) extracellular processing by proteolytic enzymes into low molecular weight fragments, of which tyrosine-rich amelogenin polypeptide (TRAP) and leucine-rich amelogenin polypeptide (LRAP) are significant because they constitute the bulk of the final organic matrix of the enamel.

Properties of Amelogenins

1. They accumulate during the secretory stage of amelogenesis.
2. They undergo minor short-term and major long-term degradation.
3. They regulate growth in thickness and width.
4. They may also nucleate crystals.

Nonamelogenins

1. *Ameloblastin* (also known as amelin or sheathlin)
   Properties:
   a. Undergoes rapid degradation.
   b. Intact molecules occur near the enamel-forming surface.
   c. Mostly fragmented forms are in deeper zones.
   d. Promotes mineral formation and crystal elongation.

2. *Enamelin*
   Properties:
   a. Undergoes small degradation in secretory stage, which decreases in deep zones, where the molecule binds with hydroxyapatite.
   b. Crystal nucleation and growth: Post-translational enamelin cleavage products bind other matrix proteins and hydroxyapatite crystals, to cause hydroxyapatite crystal growth.

3. *Sulfated glycoprotein*
   Properties: Short half-life.

4. *Tuftelin*

   It is believed to localize specifically at the dentinoenamel junction and participate in its establishment. It has been suggested to have a possible role in cell signaling. It is not specific to enamel.

At least two general classes of proteinases are involved in the extracellular processing and degradation of enamel proteins:

1. *Matrix metalloproteinase (MMP) family including MMP20 (Enamelysin):* Their function is short-term processing of newly-secreted matrix proteins.
2. *Serine proteinase 1:* Bulk digestive enzymes, particularly during the maturation stage.

The extracellular matrix of developing dental enamel is well defined in terms of its major protein components.

Forming enamel does not exhibit a distinct, unmineralized pre-enamel layer, such as osteoid or predentin, and crystals grow directly against the secretory surfaces of ameloblasts. Although, the background matrix formed by the marginally soluble amelgenins may provide some physical support, enamel proteins likely do not play any major structuring function as collagen in bone, dentin and cellular cementum. Therefore, the three-dimensional organization seen in enamel likely results from the direct organization of the extremely long crystals.

Morphologically, the organic matrix of forming enamel appears uniform in decalcified histologic preparations, however, immunohistochemical analysis has revealed that enamel proteins are differentially distributed across the enamel layer.

Intact or relatively intact nonamelogenin molecules, such as ameloblastin, are concentrated near the cell surface at sites where they are secreted, whereas mostly degradation fragments are found in deeper (older) enamel.

The sites where ameloblastin is immunodetected at the highest concentration actually correspond to particular positions in enamel where inter-rod and rod crystals grow in length. However, intact and fragmented forms of amelogenin are least concentrated at growth sites and are found abundantly throughout the enamel layer.

Amelogenin and ameloblastin are synthesized together and are contained within the same secretory granule. Their segregation at growth sites is intriguing and may result from microenvironment conditions or physicochemical properties of proteins itself.

Amelogenins are believed to form supramolecular aggregates called **nanospheres** that surround crystals along their long axis and that are visible on sections of enamel examined under the electron microscope as a granular background material between crystals. Based on the biochemical characteristics and differential distribution of the various enamel proteins, members of the nonamelogenin family are broadly believed to promote and guide the formation of enamel crystal, whereas the amelogenins regulate growth in thickness and width of crystals.

Amelogenins prevent crystals from fusing during their formation and must be removed to permit growth.

MINERALIZATION OF DENTIN

Throughout dentinogenesis, mineralization is achieved by continuous deposition of mineral, initially in the matrix vesicle and then at the mineralization front.

Odontoblasts exert control in initiating mineralization by producing matrix vesicles and proteins that can regulate mineral deposition and by adapting the organic matrix at the mineralization front so that it receives the mineral deposits.

Mineral ions reach mineralization site in dentinogenesis by a few mechanisms:

1. Junctions holding the odontoblasts together in a palisaded arrangement are incomplete and leaky. Conceptually, simple percolation of tissue fluid supersaturated with calcium and phosphate can take place.
2. Calcium channels of L type have been demonstrated in the basal plasma membrane of the odontoblast. When these channels are blocked, mineralization of dentin is affected.

The presence of alkaline phosphatase and calcium adenotriphosphatase activity at the distal end of the cell is consistent with the transport and release of mineral ions into the forming dentin layer.

References

1. Hu JCC. Enamelin and autosomal dominant amelogenesis imperfecta. Crit Rev Oral Biol Med 2003;14(6):387–98.
2. Andersen CH, Garimella Rama, Tague S. The role of matrix vesicles in growth plate development and biomineralization. Frontiers in Bioscience 2005;10(1):822–37.
3. Dziewiatkowski, DD & LL Majznerski. Role of proteoglycans in endochondral ossification: inhibition of calcification. Calcif Tissue Int 1985;37(5):560–64.
4. Lohmander, S. & A. Hjerpe. Proteoglycans of mineralizing rib and epiphyseal cartilage. Biochim Biophys Acta 1975;404(1):93–109.
5. Ortega, N, D. Behonick, D Stickens & Z. Werb: How proteases regulate bone morphogenesis. Ann N Y Acad Sci 2003;995:109–16.
6. Marino AA, Becker RO. Evidence of epitaxy in the formation of collagen and apatite. Nature 1970;226(May):652–53.

3 Calcium and Phosphate Metabolism

Calcium and phosphate metabolic physiology is a interplay of vitamin D function along with two regulatory hormones-parathyroid and calcitonin.

Functions

1. Neuromuscular excitability: Excessive calcium loss can lead to hypoirritability and vice versa
2. Blood coagulation
3. Secretory processes
4. Membrane integrity
5. Membrane transport
6. Enzyme reactions
7. Bone hardness
8. Major component of teeth.

Sources

Dairy products, beans, leafy vegetables.

Dynamics of Calcium in Human Body (Daily turnover)

	mg
Intake	1000
Intestinal absorption	350
Secretion in gastrointestinal juices	250
Net absorption over secretion	100
Loss in feces	900
Excretion in urine	100

The usual rates of intake are approximately 1 gm/day each for calcium and phosphorus. Phosphate is a "renal threshold substance", i.e. when its concentration in plasma is below the critical value of about 1 mmol/litre, no phosphate is lost into urine because all of it in glomerular filtrate is absorbed.

Role of Vitamin D in Calcium and Phosphate Metabolism

Vitamin D has a potent effect on increasing calcium absorption from the intestinal tract along with regulation of both bone deposition and reabsorption.

VITAMIN D COMPOUNDS

Vitamin D derivatives are sterols which perform more or less same functions. The most important form is Vitamin D_3 or cholecalciferol. Most of it is formed in the skin because of UV irradiation of 7-dehydrocholesterol, a naturally occurring substance in skin. Therefore, inadequate exposure to sunlight causes vitamin D deficiency.

The vitamin D compounds ingested in food are identical to cholecalciferol except for substitution of one or more atoms that do not affect their function.

Conversion of Cholecalciferol to 25-Hydroxy-cholecalciferol in Liver and its feedback Control

The first step in activation of cholecalciferol is its conversion to 25-hydroxycholecalciferol in liver. This is a limited process because the 25-hydroxycholesterol has an inhibitory feedback effect on conversion.

This feedback control is important because:

1. This regulates the precise plasma concentration of 25-hydroxycholecalciferol.
2. Conserves the vitamin D in liver for future use, as vitamin D can be stored for many months as compared to 25-hydroxycholecalciferol, which persists for only a few weeks.

Flow chart 3.1: Activation of vitamin D_3 to form 1, 25-dihydroxycholecalciferol and the role of vitamin D in controlling the plasma calcium concentration

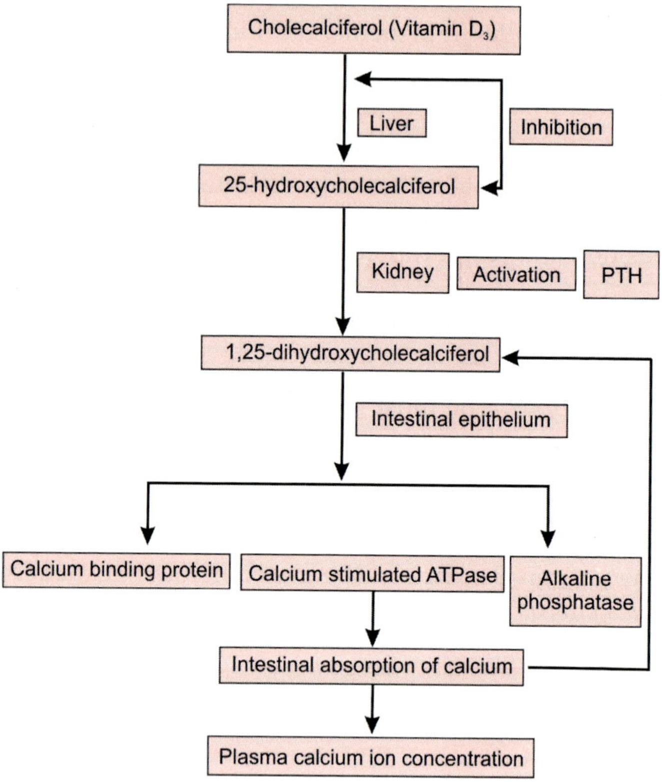

Conversion of 25-Hydroxycholecalciferol to 1, 25-Dihydroxycholecalciferol in Kidney and its Control by Parathyroid Hormone

This conversion takes place in the proximal tubules of kidney. 1, 25-dihydroxycholecalciferol is the most active form of vitamin D. Therefore, in cases of renal failure, vitamin D deficiency manifests itself. The conversion of 25-hydroxycholecalciferol to 1, 25-dihydroxycholecalciferol requires parathyroid hormone. In absence of this hormone, either none or almost none of 1, 25-dihydroxycholecalciferol is formed.

Effects of Calcium ion Concentration on Control of formation of 1, 25-Dihydroxycholecalciferol

The plasma concentration of 1, 25-dihydroxycholecalciferol is inversely proportional to the plasma calcium concentration. There are two reasons for this:

1. Calcium ion itself has a slight effect in preventing the conversion of 25-hydroxycholecalciferol to 1, 25-dihydroxycholecalciferol.
2. The rate of PTH secretion is greatly suppressed when the plasma calcium ion concentration rises above 9 to 10 mg/dl.

Therefore, at calcium concentrations below 9 to 10 mg/dl, PTH promotes the conversion of 25-hydroxycholecalciferol to 1, 25-dihydroxycholecalciferol in kidneys.

Effects of 1, 25-Dihydroxycholecalciferol on Intestinal Epithelium

1, 25-dihydroxycholecalciferol functions as a "hormone" to promote intestinal calcium absorption. This is accomplished by increasing *calcium binding protein* over a period of about two days in the intestinal epithelial cells. This protein functions in the brush borders of these cells to transport calcium into the cell cytoplasm. The calcium then moves through the basolateral cell membrane by facilitated diffusion. The rate of calcium absorption seems to be directly proportional to the quantity of this calcium binding protein. This protein remains in the cell for several weeks after 1, 25-dihydroxycholecalciferol has been removed from the body, thus prolonging its effect on calcium absorption.

Other functions of this hormone are:

1. Formation of calcium-stimulated ATPase in the brush border of epithelial cells.
2. Formation of alkaline phosphatase in epithelial cells.

Effect of Vitamin D on Phosphate Absorption

Phosphate flux through gastrointestinal epithelium is enhanced by vitamin D. This might result from:

1. Direct effect of 1, 25-dihydroxycholecalciferol.

2. Secondary to calcium absorption, with calcium acting as a transport mediator for phosphate.

Calcium in Plasma and Interstitial Fluid

The calcium concentration in plasma averages about 9.4 mg/dl, normally varying between 9 to 10 mg/dl. The calcium in plasma is present in three forms:

1. About 40% of calcium is combined with plasma proteins and is nondiffusible through capillary membrane.
2. About 10% of calcium is diffusible through the cell membrane but is nonionized due to its combination with substances like citrate and phosphate in plasma.
3. The remaining 50% of calcium in plasma is both diffusible as well as ionizable.

Inorganic Phosphate in Extracellular Fluids

Inorganic phosphate in plasma is mainly in two forms: HPO_4^{2-} and $H_2PO_4^-$. The concentration of HPO_4^{2-} is about 1.05 mmol/litre and $H_2PO_4^-$ is about 0.26 mmol/litre. When the total quantity of phosphate in the extracellular fluid rises, so does the quantity of these ionic forms.

When the pH of extracellular fluid becomes more acidic, there is a relative increase in $H_2PO_4^-$ and a decrease in HPO_4^2 whereas the opposite occurs when the extracellular fluid becomes alkaline.

Normal limits of phosphate

Adults	3–4 mg/dl
Children	4–5 mg/dl

Effects of Altered Calcium and Phosphate Concentrations in Body Fluids

a. *Hypocalcaemia:* When the extracellular fluid concentration of calcium ions falls below normal, the nervous system becomes progressively more and more excitable because this causes increased neuronal membrane permeability to sodium ions, allowing easy initiation of action potentials. At plasma calcium ion concentrations about 50% below normal, the peripheral nerve fibers become excitable enough to discharge spontaneously, initiating trains of nerve impulses that pass to peripheral skeletal muscles to elicit titanic muscle contractility, consequently resulting in tetany. Tetanic spasm in hand is termed as "Carpopedal spasm". Tetany occurs when the blood concentration of calcium falls from the normal levels of 9.4 mg/dl to about 6 mg/dl, which is only 35% below the normal calcium concentration and is lethal at about 4 mg/dl.

b. *Hypercalcemia:* When the levels of calcium in body fluids rises above normal, the nervous system is depressed and reflex activities of central nervous system become sluggish. Increased calcium ion concentration decreases the QT interval of heart and causes constipation and lack of appetite due to decreased contractility of muscle walls of gastrointestinal tract. The depressive effects of increased calcium level begin to appear when the blood calcium level rises above about 12 mg/dl, and becomes marked as calcium level rises above 15 mg/dl. When calcium level rises above 17 mg/dl in blood, calcium phosphate crystals are likely to precipitate throughout the body.

Composition of Bone

Bone is composed of:

a. *Organic matrix:* The organic matrix of bone is composed of 90–95% collagen and ground substance. The collagen fibers extend primarily along the lines of tensional force, therefore, providing tensile strength to the bone. The ground substance is composed of extracellular fluid and proteoglycans, chiefly, chondroitin sulfate and hyaluronic acid.

b. *Bone salts:* The major salt forming the bone is calcium hydroxyapatite. Its chemical formula is: $Ca_{10}\ (PO_4)_6\ (OH)_2$. Each crystal is about 400Å long, 10–30Å thick and 100Å wide and is shaped like a long, flat plate. The collagenous component of bone has great tensile strength whereas the calcium salt has great compressional strength. These combined properties provide bone with extreme tensile and compressional strength.

PARATHYROID GLANDS AND PARATHYROID HORMONE (PTH)

Parathyroid Glands

Anatomy: Normally there are four parathyroid glands in human beings, located immediately behind the thyroid gland—one behind each of the upper and lower poles, respectively. Each parathyroid gland is about 6 millimeters long, 3 millimeters wide, and 2 millimeters thick. Accidental removal of these glands during total or partial thyroidectomy might result in severe symptoms.

Removal of half of parathyroid glands usually causes little physiological abnormality. However, removal of 3 out of 4 glands usually causes transient hypoparathyroidism. Even a small quantity of remaining parathyroid tissue usually hypertrophies to perform the function of all the glands.

The adult parathyroid gland contains mainly the **chief cells** and a small to moderate number of **oxyphil cells**. The function of chief cells is to secrete PTH. The oxyphil cells are believed to be modified or depleted chief cells that do not secrete PTH.

Parathyroid Hormone (PTH)

PTH is a secretory product of parathyroid gland. This hormone is first synthesized in form of a *preprohormone*, a polypeptide chain of 110 amino acids, then, to *prohormone* with 90 amino acids and then, to *hormone* with 84 amino acids, by the endoplasmic reticulum and Golgi apparatus and finally, packaged in secretory granules in the cytoplasm of these cells. The final hormone has a molecular weight of about 9500 Daltons.

Effect of PTH on Bone

PTH has two phases on bone in causing calcium and phosphate absorption.

1. Rapid phase
2. Slow phase

Rapid phase of calcium and phosphate absorption:

Osteolysis: When large quantities of PTH are injected, the calcium ion concentration in blood begins to rise within minutes. PTH removes calcium and phosphate from two sites in bone:

a. From the bone matrix in vicinity of osteocytes
b. From the vicinity of osteoblasts

Osteoblasts and osteocytes form a system of interconnected cells that spreads all through the bone except near the osteoclasts. This extensive system is called the **osteocytic membrane system**. Between the osteocytic membrane and bone, small amount of fluid called **bone fluid** is present. The osteocytic membrane pumps calcium ions from the bone fluid into the extracellular fluid, creating a calcium ion concentration in bone fluid which is only one-third of extracellular fluid. When the osteocytic pump becomes excessively activated, the bone fluid calcium ion concentration falls even lower and calcium phosphate salts are then absorbed from the bone. This effect is called **osteolysis**. When the pump is inactivated, the bone fluid calcium ion concentration rises to a higher level and calcium phosphate salts are redeposited in the matrix. The cell membranes of both osteoblasts and osteocytes have receptor proteins for PTH.

PTH can activate the calcium pump strongly, thereby, causing rapid removal of calcium phosphate salts. The PTH is believed to stimulate this pump by increasing the calcium permeability of bone fluid side of osteocytic membrane, thus allowing calcium ions to diffuse into the membrane cells from the bone fluid. This calcium is pumped into the extracellular fluid by calcium transport system on other membrane side.

Slow phase of calcium and phosphate absorption:

This phase is characterized by activation of osteoclasts. PTH does not cause osteoclastic activation directly. It is believed that a molecular signal is sent to the activated osteoblasts and osteocytes that cause the osteoclast to function.

Activation of osteoclastic system occurs in two stages:

a. Immediate activation of already formed osteoclasts.
b. Formation of new osteoclasts.

After a few months, osteoclastic resorption leads to weakened bones (osteoporosis) and secondary stimulation of osteoblasts to correct the weakened state. Therefore, in late stages, there is more bone absorption than bone deposition in presence of excess PTH.

Effect of PTH on Kidneys

Increased PTH levels cause urinary phosphate loss owing to the diminished phosphate reabsorptive capacity from proximal tubules. At the same time, calcium absorption increases from proximal tubules along with magnesium and hydrogen ions. A decreased reabsorption of sodium, potassium and amino acid ions also occurs. Increased calcium absorption occurs mainly in the late distal tubules, collecting tubules and early collecting ducts.

Effect of PTH on Intestines

PTH greatly enhances both calcium and phosphate absorption by increasing the formation of 1, 25-dihydroxycholecalciferol from vitamin D in the kidneys.

Receptors for PTH and PTHrP (PTH related peptide)

Their biological importance and functional properties:
PTH acts primarily on kidney and bone, where it binds to cells expressing type 1 PTH/PTHrP receptor (PTH1R). PTHrP was first discovered as the most frequent cause of the syndrome of *humoral calcaemia* of malignancy. The PTHrP binds to the same receptor as PTH and the biological responses elicited are commonly indistinguishable, with regard to calcium homeostasis.

Role of PTH1R in Development

PTH1R is highly expressed in the prehypertrophic chondrocytes of metaphyseal growth plates and in these cells, mediates the autocrine/paracrine actions of PTHrP. By acting through the Wnt and BMP family of proteins, PTHrP slows the differentiation of growth plate chondrocytes and prevents them from entering the hypertrophic stage thereby, allowing the bone to grow and elongate normally.

PTHrP and PTH1R have been shown to regulate branching morphogenesis in mammary glands and also a role suggested in the development of skin, hair and teeth development.

THYROID GLAND AND CALCITONIN

Calcitonin is a weak hormone, the function of which is to reduce the blood calcium ion concentration. In lower vertebrates, it is secreted by the ultimobranchial glands. These glands do not exist among humans but are incorporated into the thyroid, where they are termed **parafollicular** or **C** cells.

Calcitonin is a large polypeptide with a molecular weight of about 3400 daltons and a chain of 32 amino acids.

Function of Calcitonin on Plasma Calcium Ion Concentration

Calcitonin decreases blood calcium ion concentration rapidly, beginning within minutes after injection. Thus, the effect of calcitonin on blood calcium ion concentration is opposite to that of PTH. Calcitonin reduces plasma calcium concentration in at least two ways:

1. *Immediate effect:* There is a decrease in absorption by the osteoclasts and probably the osteolytic effect of the osteocytic membrane. The net result is deposition of calcium in exchangeable bone calcium salts.
2. *Prolonged effect:* Long-term effect manifests as a decrease in formation of osteoclasts.

Calcitonin also acts on calcium absorption in kidneys and intestinal tract.

Applied Physiology of Parathyroid Glands

1. *Hypoparathyroidism:* Insufficient secretion of PTH results in decrease in osteocytic reabsorption of exchangeable calcium

with a decrease in osteoclastic activity. Net result is the decrease in plasma calcium level. Sudden removal of parathyroid gland results in fall in calcium level from 9.4 mg/dl to 6–7 mg/dl within two to three days and a rise in blood phosphate concentration. At this calcium concentration, signs and symptoms of tetany develop with involvement of all muscles of body, especially the laryngeal muscles, resulting in respiratory obstruction and even redundant death.

2. *Hyperparathyroidism:* Hyperparathyroidism is normally a consequence of tumor of parathyroid glands. This condition is more common in females as compared to men, the predisposing factor being pregnancy and lactation. In mild hyperparathyroidism, new bone is deposited rapidly to compensate for increased osteoclastic bone resorption whereas in severe hyperparathyroidism, osteoclastic absorption exceeds osteoblastic deposition.
3. *Parathyroid poisoning:* Whenever extremely high quantities of PTH are secreted, the calcium levels rise rapidly to high values along with phosphate levels. The body fluids become supersaturated with $CaHPO_4$ crystals, and begin to deposit in various areas of the body. This phenomenon is termed **Metastatic calcification**.
4. *Rickets:* Rickets occurs commonly in children and results from calcium or phosphate deficiency in extracellular fluid, usually caused by lack of vitamin D. Exposure to sunlight converts the 7-dehydrocholesterol present in the skin to vitamin D_3 which prevents rickets by promoting calcium and phosphate absorption from intestines. The plasma calcium concentration in rickets is slightly depressed in contrast to highly depressed levels of phosphate. During prolonged rickets, there is a marked compensatory increase in PTH secretion resulting in extreme osteoclastic bone resorption. This causes an elevation in calcium levels but a rapid rise in phosphate levels. In the early stages, there is an increase in osteoblastic activity resulting in bone deposition. However, in later stages, excessive osteoblastic activity results in exuberant osteoid deposition. Therefore, the bone formed is weak, uncalcified and immature.

5. *Osteomalacia:* Adult rickets is known as **osteomalacia** and is a result of dietary vitamin D deficiency. This deficiency may be a consequence of steatorrhea, where excessive loss of vitamin D and calcium takes place.
6. *Renal rickets:* Renal rickets is a type of osteomalacia that results from prolonged kidney damage. This results mainly due to the failure of kidneys to synthesize 1,25-dihydroxycholecalciferol (active form of vitamin D).
7. *Congenital hypophosphatemia:* This results from congenitally reduced reabsorption of phosphates by the renal tubules. This type of rickets is treated by phosphate compounds and is termed "Vitamin D-resistant rickets".
8. *Osteoporosis:* This disorder results from diminished bone matrix rather than from insufficient calcification. The most common causes of osteoporosis are:
   a. Lack of physical stress because of inactivity
   b. Malnutrition
   c. Vitamin C deficiency
   d. Postmenopausal lack of estrogen
   e. Old age
   f. Cushing's disease.

Mineral Exchange in Teeth

The salts of teeth, like bone, are composed of hydroxyapatite with absorbed carbonates and other ions. New salts are constantly being absorbed and deposited, specially in dentin and cementum. Very little amount of mineral is exchanged or deposited on enamel from saliva. The rate of absorption and deposition of minerals in cementum is almost equal to that of bone, whereas it is almost one-third in dentin. This can be attributed to the presence of synthesizing and absorptive cells in cementum which are absent in dentin.

Effect of Calcium and Phosphate Metabolism on Teeth

1. *Vitamin D-resistant rickets:* Teeth show markedly enlarged pulp horns. Dentin is abnormal and characterized by deposition of globular dentin, which often exhibits clefting.

Clefts may extend from pulp chamber to dentinoenamel junction (DEJ). Microclefts are seen in enamel. Pulp becomes nonvital due to bacterial contamination as a result of presence of clefts.

2. *Hypophosphatasia:* Teeth show an absence or reduction of cementum, which predisposes the teeth to an early exfoliation.
3. *Hypoparathyroidism:* Development of this condition during early stages of odontogenesis results in pitting enamel hypoplasia. Failure of tooth eruption may occur.
4. *Pseudohypoparathyroidism:* Generalized enamel hypoplasia, widened pulp chambers with intrapulpal calcifications, oligodontia, delayed eruption and blunting of root apices. The pulpal calcifications are described as "dagger shaped".

References

1. Carafoli E. Calcium pump of the plasma membrane. Physiol Rev 1991;71:129–35.
2. Garel JM. Hormonal control of calcium metabolism during the reproductive cycle in mammals. Physiol Rev 1987;67:1–10.
3. Habener JF, et al. Parathyroid hormone: Biochemical aspects of biosynthesis, secretion, action and metabolism. Physiol Rev 1984;64:985–90.
4. Guyton and Hall. Textbook of Medical Physiology; 9th edition. WB Saunders Company. Philadelphia.
5. Neville B, Damm D, Allen C, Bouquot J. Oral and Maxillofacial Pathology. 2nd edition. Saunders, Philadelphia.

4

Orofacial Pain

INTRODUCTION

Pain is defined as an unpleasant sensory and emotional experience associated with actual or potential tissue damage or described in terms of such damage.

Pain can be classified as:

- Acute or transient: Sharp and soon subsides.
- Persistent pain: Pain that lasts for a few days or few weeks can follow athletic injuries of the elbow, knee or elsewhere. Both these types of pain are protective.

  Or

Chronic pain: Persists long after the injury has apparently healed, possibly for months or years. This type of pain can be non-protective.

PERIPHERAL NERVOUS SYSTEM AND PAIN

The nerve cells whose axons innervate peripheral tissues (primary afferent sensory neurons) can be divided into three groups based on their diameters and degree of myelination, both of which influence their conduction velocity.

- *A beta fibers:* Large fibers that conduct impulses in the 30 to 70 m/s range. Most of these fibers are stimulated by light touch and very few are nociceptors, i.e. the receptors that respond to tissue damage.
- *A delta fibers:* Finely myelinated fibers that conduct impulses in the 3 to 30 m/s range, and many are nociceptors.
- *Unmyelinated afferents:* These are the most numerous type of nerve fibers and conduct impulses in 0.5 to 3.0 m/s range, and most are nociceptors.

There are distinct differences in the peripheral changes that follow tissue and nerve injury. Tissue damage results in an increased sensitivity of nociceptors at the site of injury. This is called **peripheral sensitization**. The nociceptors exhibit spontaneous activity, lowered thresholds, and increased responsiveness to subsequent noxious stimuli. The increased nociceptive activity leads inevitably to an increased barrage into the CNS, followed by functional changes in the spinal cord and brain that contributes to persistent pain. This is referred to as **actual sensitization**.

Sometimes nerves begin to behave abnormally and fire spontaneously, which can also lead to central sensitization. These changes are thought to contribute to the persistent pain of the neuropathic (nerve injury) type.

Both peripheral and central sensitization can lead to **hyperalgesia.**

Hyperalgesia is defined as an increased response to a stimulus that is normally painful.

Allodynia: Pain due to a stimulus that does not normally provoke pain is termed as allodynia. For example, the perception of pain produced by light touch after sunburn is an example of touch allodynia.

CENTRAL NERVOUS SYSTEM AND PAIN

Impulses carried by primary afferent nociceptive neurons from the face and from most of the mouth enter the brainstem via the trigeminal nerve. Nociceptive inputs are relayed through the trigeminal spinal nucleus, particularly its most caudal division called *subnucleus caudalis*. This subnucleus is also called the medullary dorsal horn because it is similar in structure to the spinal dorsal horn, which receives nociceptive signals from the rest of the body. Signals from the trigeminal nucleus ascend to higher centers, including the thalamus and cerebral cortex. The synapse between the peripheral neuron and the neuron in the subnucleus caudalis is an important site for signal processing. The information at this level is modulated by chemical mediators released from the terminals of several groups of neurons like, primary afferent neurons, neurons of the trigeminal nuclei and neurons of higher centers.

Descending projections are important because they provide the means by which cognitive, attentional and motivational aspects of the pain experience modulate transmission in pain pathways.

Orofacial Pain

Diagnostic range (American Academy of Orofacial Pain's classification of Head, Neck and Face Pain)

1. Intracranial/vascular pain
2. Neurovascular pain (primary headache)
3. Secondary headache related to disease/substance

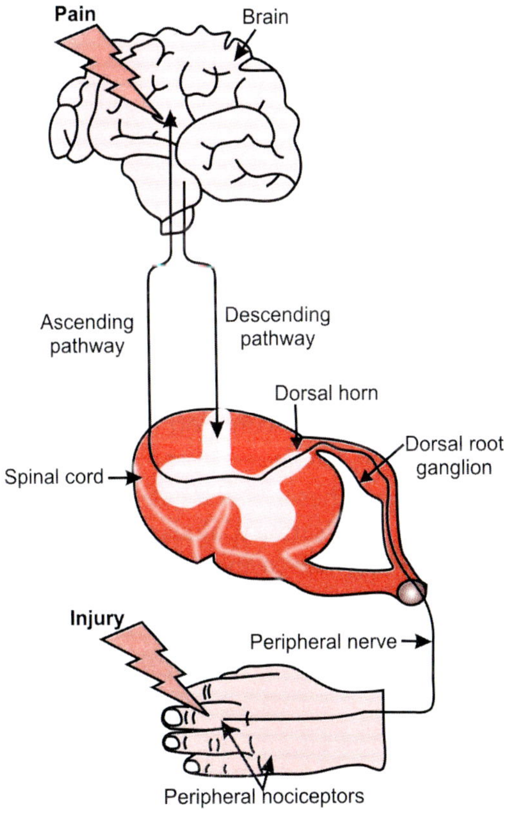

Fig. 4.1: Pain conducting ascending and descending pathways

4. Neurogenic/Neuropathic pain
5. Paroxysmal pain disorders
6. Continuous pain disorders
7. Extracranial pain disorders: Eye, ear, nose and throat.
8. Intracranial pain disorders:
   Teeth and periodontal tissues
   Mucogingival tissues
   Tongue
   Salivary glands
9. Musculoskeletal pain disorders
10. Cervical disorders
11. Temporomandibular disorders.

Intracranial Disorders

Disorders of intracranial structures, for example, neoplasm, aneurysm, abscess, hemorrhage or hematoma, can be easily differentiated from orofacial pain conditions.

a. *Neurovascular disorders (primary headache):* Neurovascular disorders associated with orofacial pain include migraine headaches, cluster headaches, chronic paroxysmal hemicrania.

   Migraine headache is divided into:
   1. Migraine with aura (classic)
   2. Migraine without aura (common migraine)
   3. Tension–type headaches

Migraine with aura: These headaches are characterized by one-sided, throbbing (pulsating) pain lasting 4 to 72 hours with frequent accompanying nausea and/or vomiting, phonophobia and photophobia. They typically have a prodomal phase with visual aberrations.

Migraine without aura: This is similar to classic migraine but proceeds into headache without prodamata.

Tension-type headaches: A type of chronic or episodic migraine-like headache. They are bilateral, mild to moderate in intensity, and characterized by a nonpulsating, pressing or tightening feeling in the head.

b. *Secondary headache:* These are secondary to another condition. These include physical exertion, cold stimuli, trauma, infection, metabolic disorders, or drug use on withdrawal. Orofacial pain is commonly associated with secondary headache.

Extracranial Pain Disorders

Neuropathic pain: Neuropathic pain is defined as pain initiated or caused by a primary lesion or dysfunction in the peripheral nervous system. Neuropathic pain disorders are divided into:

a. Paroxysmal
b. Continuous.

The paroxysmal conditions associated with orofacial pain include the following: Trigeminal neuralgia, glossopharyngeal neuralgia, superior laryngeal neuralgia, and occipital neuralgia.

The pain sensations follow the distribution of the involved nerve and are characterized by brief electric shock-like (lancinating or jabbing) pains lasting only seconds to minutes with pain-free intervals.

The continuous neuropathic pain disorders associated with orofacial pain are syndromes characterized by compression or distortion, demyelination, infarction, or inflammation of the cranial nerves.

Eye, Nose and Throat Pain

Extracranial pain disorders associated with orofacial pain include pain related to the eyes, ears, nose, sinuses, throat, intraoral structures, neck, jaw and cranial bone. The site of pain in the head, neck and orofacial region is often not the primary source of pain, making differential diagnosis extremely difficult. Referral of pain from one structure to another is common and is explained in part by the convergence of noxious input in the trigeminal spinal nucleus.

Pain in and around the eyes is relatively common, but seldom is it a result of noxious stimuli originating in the eye, extraocular muscles, or optic nerve. Rather, it is usually referred to the eye from other structures.

Pain referred to the face and mouth from the eye is infrequent, but is frequent from the ear in conditions such as otitis media and externa, mastoiditis, eustachian tube disorders, and neoplasias.

Pain in the nose and paranasal sinuses can arise from inflammation, infection and malignant disease, but pathology in these structures can cause referred pain in adjacent structures, such as the teeth.

Due to broad sensory innervation of throat, pain is referred to and from both adjacent and distant structures.

International Headache Society's Classification and Diagnostic Criteria for Headache Disorders, Cranial Neuralgias and Facial Pain

11th classification for headache or facial pain associated with extracranial structures

- Cranial bones including the mandible
- Neck
- Eyes
- Nose and sinuses
- Teeth and related oral structures
- Temporomandibular joint.

Intraoral Pain

Intraoral pain includes odontogenic pain and pain associated with the mucogingival tissues, tongue and salivary glands.

a. *Odontogenic pain:* It is defined as pain associated with the teeth and periodontium. It includes reversible pulpitis, irreversible pulpitis and pulpal necrosis. Pain is often referred to other teeth as well as to distant areas in the head, neck and jaw. Pain conditions associated with the supporting tissues of the teeth include acute apical periodontitis, acute apical abscess, and acute periodontal abscess.

b. *Mucogingival and glossal pain disorders:* These are of two types: Localized and Generalized.

   Localized pain conditions: Acute Necrotizing Ulcerative Gingivitis (ANUG), recurrent aphthous stomatitis (RAS), herpes simplex, candidiasis and injury from trauma.

Generalized pain conditions: Chemotherapy, radiation therapy, dermatologic disorders, and systemic disease including pain secondary to HIV.

c. *Musculoskeletal pains:* These are major causes of nonodontogenic pain in the orofacial region. They include- cervical spine and TMJ (articular) disorders and cervical muscle and masticatory disorders.

d. *Temporomandibular disorders*

American Academy of Orofacial Pain's Classification of Temporomandibular Disorders

1. *Masticatory muscle disorders*
   - Myofascial pain
   - Myositis
   - Myospasm or trismus
   - Local myalgia–unclassified
   - Myofibrotic contracture
   - Neoplasia.
2. *Articular disorders*
   - Congenital or developmental disorders
   - Disc derangement disorders
   - Temporomandibular dislocation
   - Inflammatory disorders
   - Osteoarthritis
   - Ankylosis
   - Fracture.

Neurobiology of Pain

Peripheral Mechanisms of Orofacial Pain

The orofacial tissues are innervated almost exclusively by branches of the trigeminal (V) sensory nerve. The V primary afferent fibers terminate in these tissues in sense organs (receptors) that are quite complex in their structure, and respond to tactile stimulation, e.g. low-threshold mechanoreceptors or to propioceptive stimuli such as stretch or tension (e.g. proprioceptors).

Other primary afferents may terminate as free nerve endings, many of which respond to noxious stimuli and these are called **nociceptors**. These so-called nociceptive afferents are generally small-diameter, myelinated and are slow conducting than A-beta and A-delta afferents that convey tactile or propioceptive information into the CNS.

The nociceptive afferents convey sensory information as action potentials from the nociceptors into the CNS and thereby provide the brain with sensory discriminative information about spatial and temporal qualities of the noxious stimuli.

Localization of stimulus occurs by the **receptive field** of the fiber, i.e. the area of skin, mucosa or deep tissue from which the afferent fiber and its associated receptors can be excited by a threshold stimulus. The area of a receptive field of a nociceptive afferent fiber is usually <1 mm^2, and the threshold for its excitation from the receptive field is very high and in noxious range.

Nociceptive stimuli particularly in the superficial tissues also activate other receptors such as mechanoreceptors that code for touch, and thus, play an important role in determining the location and quality of sensation perceived.

In tissues that have no touch receptors, such as tooth pulp and muscles, nociceptive stimuli give rise to different quality of pain sensation.

Tissue damage produced by the noxious stimulus causes the release of chemical mediators from surrounding tissues (e.g. prostaglandin, bradykinins) that activate nerve endings. Their activation may result in the production of action potentials in the A-delta and/or C fiber afferents, which are conveyed into the CNS and may elicit the perception of transient or acute pain.

Substances synthesized in and released from the afferent fibers themselves may influence the excitability of nociceptive afferents. For example, neurotrophins such as nerve growth factor and neuropeptides such as substance P and calcitonin gene related peptide (CGRP).

Neurotransmitters such as noradrenaline released from sympathetic efferents innervating the tissues may also modulate the excitability of nociceptors.

In some situations, the tissue damage may lead to abnormal nerve changes that are associated with so-called **ectopic** or **aberrant neural discharges**.

Increased excitability of the nociceptors may occur at the site of injury in many cases of tissue damage or inflammation. This is termed **nociceptor** or **peripheral sensitization**.

The processes and chemical mediators involved in producing peripheral sensitization include the products of tissue injury as well as the release of neurochemicals (e.g. neuropeptides such as substance P and CGRP) that are synthesized in the primary afferent cell bodies of nociceptive afferents and are released from the afferent endings. These neuropeptides may cause platelets, mast cells, macrophages and other cells of immune system to release inflammatory mediators such as histamine, serotonin, bradykinins and cytokines. Release of neuropeptides and these inflammatory mediators result in cardinal signs of inflammation, i.e. edema, redness, and local rise in temperature. This process has been termed **neurogenic inflammation**, because the origin is from nerves.

These chemicals also act on the nociceptive afferent endings and contribute to the peripheral sensitization. Sensitized nociceptors exhibit spontaneous activity, lowered activation thresholds, and increased responsiveness to noxious stimuli.

These chemicals may also diffuse through the peripheral tissues and act on the endings adjacent to nociceptive afferents, and thus contribute to the size and spread of painful area. The increased afferent barrage into the CNS from increased nociceptor activity may lead to functional changes in central nociceptive processing that contribute to persistent pain.

Central processes such as central sensitization seem to be involved in so-called **secondary hyperalgesia**, which refers to increased sensitivity to noxious stimuli well beyond the site of injury.

In contrast, peripheral processes involving peripheral sensitization of nociceptive afferent endings at the injury site can account for the increased pain sensitivity at the site of injury (**primary hyperalgesia**).

SPECIFIC OROFACIAL NOCICEPTIVE AFFERENTS

Dentin and Dental Pulp

Pulp is a highly vascular and richly innervated tissue that is exquisitely sensitive to stimulation. Dentin is also a sensitive tissue due to afferent fibers supplied by pulp. The nerve fibers innervating the pulp arborize extensively, especially in coronal part of tooth and form a subodontoblastic plexus.

The branches of V nerve that innervate teeth contain both afferent and postganglionic sympathetic axons. The V primary afferent neurons have their cell bodies in the trigeminal ganglion and are primarily sensory in function, although some produce vasodilatation when stimulated. This vasodilatation is part of the axon reflex pathway.

The sympathetic fibers supply the pulp vessels and are vasoconstrictor. Their cell bodies are in the superior cervical ganglion, from which the axons pass to the V ganglion and then on to the tooth in branches of V nerve.

The pulp is innervated by myelinated A-beta and A-delta fibers and nonmyelinated C fibers. About 50% of myelinated axons are of fast conducting A-beta class.

There are no axons with myelin sheaths in the odontoblastic cell layer. Some of the nerve endings contain neuropeptides, including substance P and calcitonin gene-related peptide (CGRP).

The pulp innervation is in dynamic state, and injury or ageing, for example, can be associated with changes in neurochemicals within pulp afferents as well as in the type, structure, and distribution of these afferents. For example, dentin cavity preparation can induce an increased production of nerve growth factor and sprouting of CGRP-containing nerve fiber.

Sensory Mechanisms of Dentin

Three theories have been proposed:

a. *Neural theory:* This theory attributes activation of an initial excitation of these nerve endings within the dentinal tubules that generates nerve signals, which are then conducted along the parent primary afferent nerve fibers in the pulp into the dental nerve branches and then into the brain.

b. *Hydrodynamic theory:* This theory proposes that the stimuli cause a displacement of the fluid within the dentinal tubules. The displacement occurs in either an outward or inward direction, and this mechanical disturbance is thought to activate the nerve endings in the dentin or pulp.

c. *Transduction theory:* This theory proposes that the stimuli initially excite the odontoblastic process or body, the membrane of which may come into the apposition with that of the nerve endings in the pulp or in dentinal tubules, and that the odontoblast transmits this excitation to these associated nerve endings.

Periodontal Ligament and Oral Mucous Membrane

In addition to a very dense innervation by low-threshold mechanoreceptors, the periodontal ligament contains free nerve endings. These are associated with A-delta and C-fiber nociceptive afferents that may respond to mechanical, thermal, and/or chemical stimuli. The different classes are, in general, similar to nociceptors in other tissues. Some periodontal nociceptive afferents branch to innervate the pulp of an adjacent tooth.

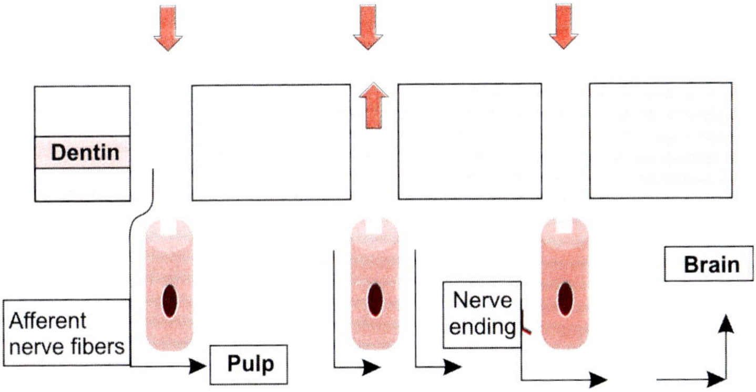

Fig. 4.2: Neural theory, hydrodynamic theory and transduction theory

Cornea

Pain appears to be the only sensation that can be evoked by stimulation of the cornea. In the cornea, the receptors are exposed to changes in the external environment. The nerve terminals penetrate into the corneal epithelium and respond to a wide range of mechanical, thermal, and chemical stimuli, all of which cause pain in humans. They have a low pain threshold, which is usually less than nociceptors in skin.

Facial Skin

The cutaneous tissues of the orofacial region have a dense innervation, especially in the perioral region. Three major classes of nociceptive afferent fibers are present:

a. *A-delta mechanothermal nociceptive afferents:* These respond to intense thermal and mechanical stimuli.

b. *C nociceptive afferents:* These are excited by strong mechanical, thermal and chemical stimuli.

c. *High threshold mechanoreceptive afferents:* These respond to intense mechanical stimuli.

Temporomandibular Joint and Masticatory Muscles

The available literature on small-diameter TMJ and masticatory muscle afferents is limited. However, the spinal afferent small diameter endings respond to a wide range of peripheral stimuli, e.g. heavy pressure, inflammatory agents.

CENTRAL NOCICEPTIVE PATHWAYS

Afferent Inputs and Brainstem Organizational Features

Most primary afferents innervating cutaneous, intraoral, deep (e.g. joint, muscle) and cerebrovascular tissues have their cell bodies in the trigeminal ganglion and project centrally to the V ganglion and project centrally to the V brainstem sensory nuclear complex, where they may ascend or descend in the V spinal tract.

In the tract, they give off collaterals that terminate in one or more subdivisions of the V brainstem sensory nuclear complex

Flow chart 4.1: Events leading to the production of central sensitization of central nociceptive neurons by peripheral injury or inflammation

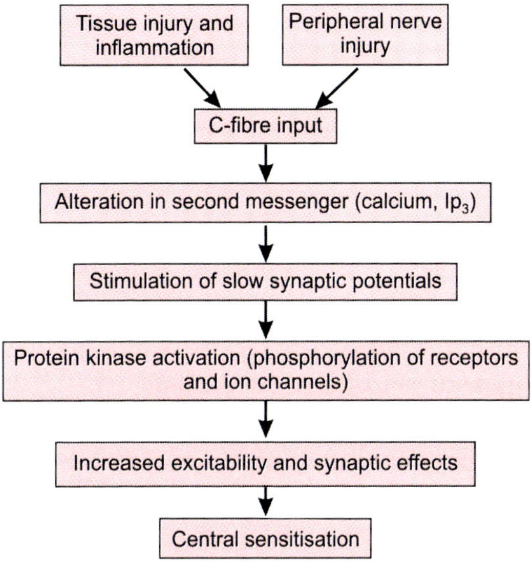

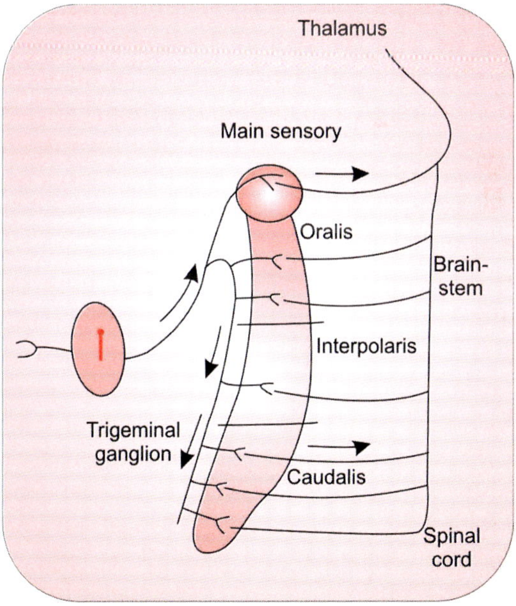

Fig. 4.3: Major somatosensory pathway from mouth and face

and activate second-order neurons within or adjacent to this V brainstem complex.

In addition to V afferent inputs, the trigeminal brainstem complex receives afferent inputs from other cranial nerves, as well as from upper cervical nerves which also send afferent inputs from other cranial nerves, as well as from upper cervical nerves which also send afferent inputs into the upper cervical dorsal horn.

Some V afferents may project to other parts of the brainstem (e.g. the solitary tract nucleus, reticular formation, supratrigeminal nucleus).

The brainstem complex can be subdivided into:

1. The main or principal sensory nucleus
2. The spinal tract

The spinal tract nucleus comprises three subnuclei: Oralis, interpolaris and caudalis.

Subnucleus caudalis is a laminated structure resembling the dorsal horn of the spinal cord; it extends into the cervical spinal cord where it merges with the spinal dorsal horn.

Neurons in the V spinal brainstem complex are somatotopically arranged. Most neurons in the dorsal part of each component receive mandibular primary afferent inputs and have receptive fields within the craniofacial region supplied by the mandibular branch of the V nerve (A neuronal receptive field is that portion of the body which, when stimulated at threshold, excites the neuron).

The ventral part contains neurons receiving ophthalmic primary afferent inputs and having an ophthalmic receptive field.

The maxillary region is represented in the area between dorsal and ventral parts. The oral and perioral structures are usually represented medially, e.g. tooth pulp primary afferents predominantly terminate on neurons in medial aspects of the nuclei and subnuclei, with upper and lower teeth represented in a mediolateral sequence and projections from anterior to posterior teeth organized in a ventrolateral to dorsolateral sequence.

In subnucleus caudalis, however, this inverted medially facing pattern of representation of the face and mouth may shift, such that receptive fields in the perioral region are found in the rostral part of the subnucleus and receptive fields in the more lateral regions of the face more caudally. This particular somatotropic pattern in subnucleus caudalis has been referred to as an "Onion-skin" arrangement.

Brainstem Nociceptive Transmission

Involvement of Trigeminal Subnucleus Caudalis

Subnucleus caudalis is the principal brainstem relay site of V nociceptive information. For example, transection of the V spinal tract (V tractomy) at the rostral pole of subnucleus caudalis for the relief of excruciating pain of trigeminal neuralgia produces a marked reduction in perception of noxious stimuli applied to the face.

The small diameter (A delta and C fiber) afferents carrying nociceptive information from the various craniofacial tissues predominantly terminate in caudalis, in its laminae I, II V and VI. In contrast, the A fiber primary afferents conducting low-threshold mechanosensitive (tactile) information terminate primarily in the more rostral components of the V brainstem complex and in laminae III to VI of caudalis. These neurons have been categorized as:

1. Nociceptive specific (NS)
2. Wide dynamic range (WDR)

The NS neurons respond only to noxious stimuli applied to a localized receptive field and receive small-diameter afferent inputs from A-delta and/or C fibers.

The WDR neurons receive both large and small diameter A fiber inputs that transmit non-noxious (e.g. tactile) information.

Both NS and WDR neurons increase their firing frequency progressively as the intensity of noxious stimulation is gradually increased or as more of receptive field is stimulated.

All nuclei and subnuclei of V brainstem complex contain low-threshold mechanoreceptive neurons that are responsive to light stimulation of a localized receptive field in the facial skin or mouth, but not noxious stimuli.

The central endings of V nociceptive primary afferents within caudalis contain certain excitatory amino acids (e.g. glutamate) and neuropeptides (e.g. substance P, calcitonin gene related peptide) that transmit the nociceptive signals to the second-order V nociceptive neurons.

In lamina II of caudalis, i.e. substantia gelatinosa, the axons of most SG neurons arborize locally within the V brainstem complex and release neuromodulatory substances like enkephalin or GABA (Gamma Aminobutyric Acid).

The substantia gelatinosa receives a mix of inputs from other areas in the brain as well as craniofacial afferent inputs, and is one of the main sites by which peripheral afferent and brain centers modulate somatosensory transmission.

Noxious craniofacial stimulation results in release of substance P within caudalis, presumably from the nociceptive afferent terminals within the subnucleus, and the released substance P acts through neurokinin receptors to produce a long-latency, sustained excitation of the nociceptive neurons that can be blocked by substance P antagonists.

Mechanism of Neuropathic Pain Central Sprouting

Peripheral injury may be associated with morphologic modifications at the central endings of the primary afferent fibers.

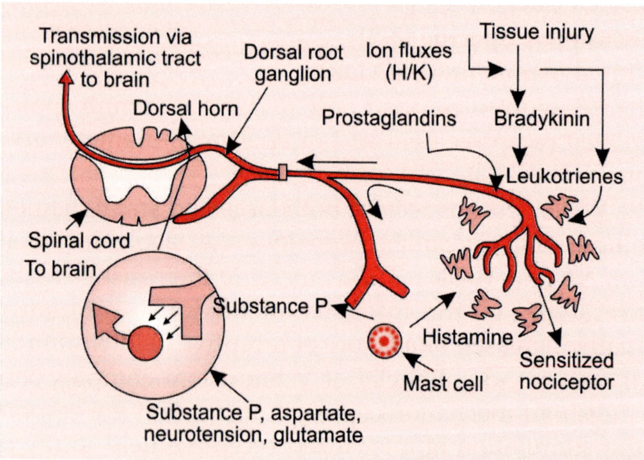

Fig. 4.3: Pain neurochemistry

Section of peripheral nerve results in reorganization of the central branching of axonal endings of A-beta primary afferents. After sprouting, the terminals that were previously distributed in layers III and IV of spinal dorsal horn make synaptic contacts in more superficial layers of the dorsal horn. This would explain some types of allodynia if the terminals of A-beta afferents that transmit tactile messages were to make contact with nociceptive neurons present in these superficial layers.

Phenotypical Changes in Primary Afferents and Dorsal Horn Neurons

One of the well-known mechanisms of pain following a nerve injury is the recognition of long-term alterations in gene expression.

Phenotypical modifications include an increase or decrease in metabolic synthesis within neurons of ionic channel proteins, neurotransmitters, neuromodulators, neurotrophins, and their receptors.

In response to axonal injury, primary afferent neurons often show electrophysiological changes by developing or increasing the baseline level of spontaneous activity or by developing high-frequency bursts of action potentials.

Abnormal expression of sodium channel genes is one of the best-documented explanations of signs of neuropathic pain. Many sodium channels with different properties exist, and nerve injury can modify, increase or decrease the expression of some of these channels. As a result, some sodium channels accumulate near the injured membrane of nociceptive primary afferents. This probably leads to an increased sodium conductance, which in turn participates in the neuronal hyperexcitability.

A sodium conductance increase also strongly contributes to the mechanisms of ectopic impulses. In neuropathic conditions, expression of excitatory neurochemicals such as substance P and CGRP is decreased, although it is increased during inflammation.

Changes in Segmental Inhibitory Control

At the V and spinal dorsal horn levels, input from A-beta afferent fibers normally controls the transmission of input from A-beta and C fibers to pain pathways.

Pain occurs when the inhibitory influence of large-fiber input is reduced or when small-fiber afferent input is increased in such a way that imbalance between them is created. Segmental inhibitory control acts through inhibitory interneurons. It has been proposed that large amounts of excitatory amino acids are released after sensory nerve injury. The alterations or destruction of these inhibitory interneurons would lead to the development of hyperexcitability of the postsynaptic V or spinal neurons.

A section of pulpal nerves associated with endodontic therapy causes degeneration-like alterations in the central endings of V primary afferents and in second-order neurons. A prolonged impairment of neuronal properties in the V brainstem complex has been noted after endodontic approaches.

The loss of segmental inhibitory control may result in the recruitment of normally ineffective synapses. The edge of the receptive field of individual V or spinal neurons is regulated by inhibitory or relatively ineffective synapses forming a

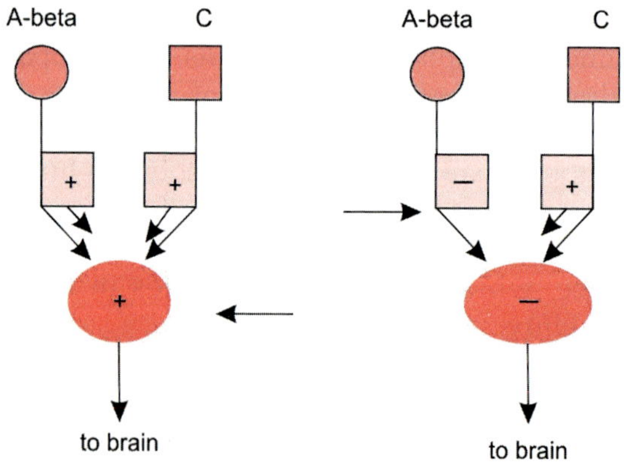

Fig. 4.4: Diagrammatic representation between excitatory and inhibitory influences

subliminal fringe. This implies that some afferents contact the central neuron under consideration but the corresponding synapse may be either insufficiently powerful to induce an excitatory effect or be counterbalanced by an ongoing inhibitory influence.

I. Normal transmission of nociception in the ascending pathways originating from the wide dynamic range of neurons. Inhibitory interneurons (in green) are triggered by activity in the large-diameter (A-beta) afferent fibers and limit the influence of the excitatory input from A and C fibers.

II. Persistent pain resulting from loss of inhibitory interneurons.

APPLIED ORAL PAIN PHYSIOLOGY

Trigeminal Neuralgia (Tic douloureux and Fothergill's disease)

Trigeminal neuralgia is an archetype of orofacial neuralgias following the anatomical distribution of trigeminal or fifth cranial nerve.

Etiology

1. *Odontogenic:* The proximity of teeth to the site of pain might have led to the postulation of its odontogenic origin. However, countless number of extractions have ruled out its odontogenic origin.
2. Periodontal origin.
3. Traumatic occlusion.
4. Compression of trigeminal roots by tumors or vascular anomalies.
5. Abnormal vessels, aneurysms, tumors, chronic meningeal inflammation.
6. An area of demyelination, as seen in multiple sclerosis.
7. Idiopathic.

Clinical Features

Older adults are mainly affected (before 35 years of age) with female predilection (3:2). It mainly affects the second and third divisions of the trigeminal nerve and always exhibits a trigger zone, stimulation of which initiates paroxysms of pain. The pain is often accompanied by a brief facial spasm or tic. Pain distribution is unilateral and lasts for few seconds to a minute.

Differential Diagnosis

1. *Horner's syndrome:* This type of headache or pain can be persistent, over a period of hours and has "no trigger zone".
2. *Sinusitis:* This can be excluded by clinical aspects of trigeminal neuralgia.
3. Costen syndrome.
4. Nasopharyngeal masses.
5. Postherpetic neuralgia.

Paratrigeminal Syndrome (Raeder's syndrome, paratrigeminal neuralgia)

It is a disease characterized by severe headache or pain in the area of the trigeminal distribution with signs of ocular sympathetic paralysis.

Auriculotemporal Syndrome (Frey's syndrome, gustatory sweating)

This syndrome arises as a result of damage to the Auriculotemporal nerve and subsequent reinnervation of sweat glands by parasympathetic salivary fibers.

Etiology

This syndrome follows surgical removal of a parotid tumor or ramus of mandible, or parotitis. As the damaged nerve regenerates, the parasympathetic nerve supply develops to salivary glands. This nerve supply then responds to salivary, gustatory or psychic stimulation.

Clinical features

Patients typically exhibits flushing and sweating of the involved side of the face, chiefly in temporal area, during eating.

References

1. Lund JP, Lavigne GJ. Orofacial pain. Quintessence Publishing Co.
2. Miles T, Narentofte B, Svensson P. Clinical Oral Physiology. Quintessence Publishing Co.
3. Behrman S. Facial neuralgias. Br Dent J 1949;86:197–206.
4. Bohn E, Strang RR. Glossopharyngeal neuralgia. Brain 1962;85: 371–74.

5

Free Radicals and Antioxidants

INTRODUCTION

A free radical is any species capable of independent existence containing one or more unpaired electrons. Examples of free radicals are: Superoxide(O_2^{2-}), thiyl(RS), trichloromethyl (CCl_3^-), and nitric oxide ($NO^\cdot$) radicals.

A free radical works in numerous ways:

1. *Electron donation:*

   $x^\cdot + y \rightarrow y^- + x^+$

2. *Electron removal:*

   $x^\cdot + y \rightarrow y^- + x^-$

3. *Addition:*

   $x^\cdot + y^\cdot \rightarrow (x—y)^\cdot$

   Only when two free radicals meet, a chain reaction, which results in formation of more free radicals, is terminated.

$$x^\cdot + y^\cdot \rightarrow xy$$

Free Radicals in Vivo

Free radicals and other reactive oxygen species are continuously produced *in vivo*. This has resulted in development of anti-oxidant mechanisms within organisms.

a. *Hydroxyl radical:* Hydroxyl radicals are produced in living organisms by at least two mechanisms:

   1. Reaction of transition metals with hydrogen peroxide.
   2. Homolytic fusion of water caused by exposure to ionizing radiation.

      Hydroxyl radicals are a reactive species that can attack all biologic molecules, usually setting off free radical chain reaction.

b. *Superoxide radical:* Superoxide radical is much less reactive than OH^-. O_2^{2-} reacts with nitric oxide, a free radical produced by several cell types (especially, phagocytes and vascular endothelial cells) to produce peroxynitrite.

Nitric oxide, or a derivative of it, acts on smooth muscle cells in vessel walls to produce relaxation. By opposing its action, therefore, O_2^{2-} can act as a vasoconstrictor and can thus, have deleterious effects in some clinical situations.

Some of the O_2^{2-} production that occurs is the result of auto-oxidation reactions and the "leakage" of electrons from electron transport chain.

Removal of excess O_2^{2-} by superoxide dismutase (SOD) enzymes is an important antioxidant defense mechanism in aerobic organisms. SOD enzymes convert O_2^{2-} into O_2 and H_2O_2. H_2O_2 acts as a metabolic signal under certain circumstances, possibly by oxidizing specific protein thiol groups triggering intracellular events. For example, H_2O_2 can cause expression of HIV genes in infected cells, possibly by oxidizing the nuclear regulatory protein, NF-κβ.

H_2O_2 crosses cell membranes easily and it can attack, apparently directly, a few cellular targets. For example, high levels of H_2O_2 can inactivate the glycolytic enzyme, glyceraldehyde-3-phosphate dehydrogenase.

Transition Metals

Transition metals usually promote free radical reactions. For example, several transition metal salts reduce H_2O_2 in a one – electron reaction to generate OH^-.

$$M^{n+} + H_2O_2 \rightarrow M^{(n+1)+} + OH^{\cdot} + OH^-$$

Where M^{n+} may be Ti (III), Cu (I), Fe(II), Co(II), or Ni(II).

$$Ti(III) + H_2O_2 \rightarrow Ti\ (IV) + OH + OH^-$$

Fenton Reaction

Ferrous salts react with H_2O_2 to form OH^- by the so-called Fenton reaction,

$$Fe(II) + H_2O_2 \rightarrow Fe\ (III) + OH + OH^-$$

Thus, the initial product of the above reaction may be an oxo-iron complex, possibly ferryl, that decomposes to form OH

$$Fe(II) + H_2O_2 \rightarrow FeOH^{3+} \text{ (or } FeO^{2+}) \rightarrow Fe\text{ (III)} + OH \quad (1)$$

Different ligands to iron (II) may stabilize this intermediate reaction, so that little OH^- is formed. Iron-ethylenediaminetetraacetic acid chelates are good sources of OH^- in the presence of H_2O_2 whereas, heme rings appear to stabilize ferryl species.

Reducing agents like ascorbate can also stimulate Fenton reaction,

$$Fe(III) + \text{Ascorbate} \rightarrow Fe(II) + \text{semidehydroascorbate}$$

Hence, iron salt-ascorbate-H_2O_2 mixtures are good sources of $OH^\cdot$ radical. Superoxide can reduce certain ferric chelates. Reaction of Fe(III) with O_2^- appears to proceed via a perferryl intermediate.

$$Fe\text{ (III)} + O_2^- \rightarrow Fe^{3+} - O_2 \longleftrightarrow Fe^{2+} - O_2 \longleftrightarrow Fe^{2+} + O_2 \quad (2)$$

The sum of reactions 1 and 2 is:

$$O_2^- + H_2O_2 \xrightarrow{Fe^{3+}} OH^- + OH^- + O_2$$

This reaction is often called the iron-catalyzed **Haber-Weiss reaction**, or the superoxide-driven Fenton reaction and appears to account for at least part of the damage that is caused to living cells by excess generation of ROS and can be inhibited by several iron-chelating agents. For example, desferoxamine.

Nonpharmacological/Natural Antioxidant Defense Mechanisms

Antioxidant defense mechanisms include enzymes (superoxide dismutase, catalase, glutathione peroxidases) and the safe sequestration of transition metal ions. Many physiologic antioxidants act by scavenging radicals.

1. *Tocopherols:* Tocopherols delay lipid peroxidation by scavenging intermediate radicals such as lipid peroxyls.

Tocopherols function by transferring a hydrogen atom with its single electron and thus, removing the peroxyl free radical.

$$\text{Lipid} - O_2^- + \text{tocopherol} - OH \rightarrow \text{lipid-}O_2H + \text{tocopherol}$$

2. *Ascorbic acid:* Ascorbic acid has a multiplicity of antioxidant properties and is the most important antioxidant in human plasma, partly because of the reason that it usually disappears faster than other antioxidants when plasma gets exposed to reactive oxygen species (ROS) produced during oxidative stress. The ability of ascorbate to show antioxidant properties is related to its fast reaction with many ROS (especially peroxyl radicals) and to the fact that the resulting semidehydroascorbate radical is poorly reactive.

		Increase in radical-generating enzymes (e.g. xanthine oxidase)
		Activation of phagocytes
Heat		Activation of phospholipases, cyclooxygenases and lipooxygenases
Radiation	Tissue damage	
Trauma		Destruction of antioxidants
Ultrasound		Release of "free" metal ions
Infection		
Hypoxia		Release of heme proteins
Toxins		Disruption of electron transport chain and increased electron leakage to form O_2^-
Exercise		

3. *Glutathione:* Glutathione is an important substrate for glutathione peroxidases, transferases, and several other enzymes and acts as a general *radical scavenger* in cells. It might also help to recycle tocopherol radicals *in vivo* in both cases by donating its hydrogen atom.

Pharmacologically Derived Antioxidants

1. *ACE inhibitors:* Captopril, an angiotensin converting enzyme inhibitor is a free radical scavenger due to the presence of sulphydryl group in the molecule.
2. *Calcium channel blockers:* Nifedipine and Verapamil act by suppression of lipid peroxidation and enhance recovery of myocardial contractility in experimental rats' hearts.
3. *Pentoxyfilline:* This drug blocks cytokine-induced leukocyte adherence chemotaxis and free radical production.
4. *Gabexate mersilate:* It is a leukocyte adhesion inhibitor and has been recommended for free radical-induced disorders such as endotoxin shock, acute pancreatitis and polyarthritis. This drug acts as a free radical scavenger by inhibiting superoxide production by neutrophils.
5. *Desferrioxamine:* This drug acts by preventing formation of hydroxyl free radicals by chelating iron and copper. It is used for management of rheumatoid arthritis.

Management of Oral Diseases with Antioxidants

a. *Oral cancer and pre-cancer:* DNA is the main target of free radical damage. The types of damages induced include strand breaks, base damage, damage to deoxyribose sugar as well as DNA protein cross-links. These damages can result in mutations that cause changes in protooncogenes and tumor suppressor genes leading to carcinogenesis. Experimental and epidemiological data indicate a therapeutic role of antioxidants like vitamins A, C, E, beta-carotene and micronutrients. Low intake of carotenoids has been related to high cancer risk. Smokers have lower beta-carotene levels in plasma and mucosal cells than non-smokers.

   Chemotherapeutic phytochemicals can block initiation or reverse the promotion stage of multistep carcinogenesis. They can also stop or retard the progression of precancerous cells to malignant ones. Intracellular signal transduction pathways converge with the activation of transcription factors, NF-κβ. As these factors mediate pleiotropic effects of both external and internal stimuli in cellular signaling cascades, they are the prime targets of chemopreventive phytochemicals.

b. *Chronic (Idiopathic) orofacial pain:* In a study on patients diagnosed with chronic facial pain as in conditions like facial arthromyalgia, TMJ dysfunction syndrome, high intra-articular concentrations of hyperalgesic mediator, 15-hydroxyl eicosatetraenoic acid (15-HETE) have been demonstrated. Synthesis of 15-HETE involves free radical-mediated process of lipid peroxidation of arachidonic acid in synovial fluid. Use of anti-oxidants help alleviate symptoms due to scavenging of free radicals.

Conclusion

Free radicals are products of normal metabolic processes as well as of external agents like drugs and radiation. Production of free radicals is counterbalanced by antioxidants which are naturally occurring as well as synthetically produced.

References

1. Ansari KN. The free radicals—The hidden culprits – An update. Ind J of Med Sci1997;51(9):319–36.
2. Devasagayam TPA, Tilak JC, Boloor KK, Sane KS, Ghaskabdi SS, Lele RD. Free radicals and antioxidants in human health: Current status and future prospects. JAPI 2004 Oct;52:794–03.
3. Halliwell B. Free radicals, antioxidants, and human disease: curiosity, cause or consequences. The Lancet 1994 Sept; 344(10):721–24.
4. Halliwell B, Gutteridge JM and Cross CE. Free radicals, antioxidants, and human disease: Where are we now? J Lab Clin Med 1992 June; 119(6):598–62.

6

Taste

In most air-breathing vertebrates, chemosensitivity is divided into a contact chemical sense called taste and a distant chemical sense called smell. In taste sensation, chemicals in solution are brought into contact with the chemoreceptors whereas, in olfaction, the chemicals are carried to the chemoreceptors as vapors in inspired air.

Taste Receptors

Mammalian taste buds are widely distributed throughout the oral cavity, pharynx and larynx. Most lingual taste buds are confined to the dorsal and lateral borders of the tongue and are associated with specialized structures called papillae.

There are four main types of papillae: Filiform, fungiform, circumvallate and foliate.

The most numerous are the filiform papillae, located over the anterior and posterior dorsum, which do not contain taste buds and therefore, have no gustatory function.

The fungiform papillae contain one or more taste buds on their upper surface and are confined to the anterior two-thirds of the tongue. There are large numbers of fungiform papillae, about 200 in the humans.

The circumvallate papillae are found at the junction of the oral and pharyngeal parts of the tongue. Taste buds are located on the sides of the papillae and sometimes, in the wall surrounding the papillae.

The foliate papillae are found on the posterior, lateral border of the tongue and consist of a series of folds forming clefts on the tongue surface. Taste buds are found in the epithelium of the cleft walls.

Tongue is not the only site where taste buds are found. Significant numbers of them are found on the palate and larynx. In these locations, the taste buds are not contained on specialized papillae but are distributed in the surface epithelium.

Structure

Taste buds are goblet-shaped structures spanning the depth of the epithelium in which they are situated. Each bud consists of about 50 spindle-shaped, modified, epithelial cells that extend from the basement membrane to the epithelial surface. At the epithelial surface, the tapered apical ends of the taste buds are in contact with the fluid environment of the oropharynx and larynx through a narrow channel called the taste pore. Terminal branches of gustatory nerve fibers enter the taste buds at its base and distribute among the taste cells. Synaptic transmission occurs between the taste bud cells and gustatory nerve terminals.

Ultrastructural examination of taste buds has revealed that they contain a number of different cell types based on morphological features. Not all cells can be unequivocally categorized because the different cell shapes observed in formalin fixed specimens represent various stages in the life cycle of a single cell type. There are four types of taste bud cells:

Type I (dark cells)

These cells are long and narrow, extending from the base of the taste bud to taste pore. They comprise approximately 60% of the total cell population. These electron-dense cells are characterized by large dense vesicles in the apical cytoplasm and a deeply invaginated nucleus.

Type II (light cells)

These cells also extend from the basement membrane to the taste pore and are characterized by electrolucent cytoplasm and large, round or oval nuclei. These cells are less numerous than type I cells, comprising about 30% of population.

Type III

These cells have apical specializations that extend into the taste pore and are similar in morphology to type II cells.

Type IV

This cell type touches the basement membrane but does not extend to the taste pore and is called basal cell.

The initial contact between the taste stimuli and taste receptors takes place in the taste pore. Tight junctions join the apices of the taste bud cells at the base of the pore, effectively separating the external environment of the oral cavity and the internal environment below the tight junctions of oral cavity.

Nerve fibers enter the taste buds by penetrating the basal lamina. Within the taste bud, the nerve processes branch, widen, and narrow again to contact other nerve processes. These nerve fibers make ill-defined contacts with the taste bud cells. This primitive nature of contact between taste cells and nerve fibers is due to the short life cycle of taste cells.

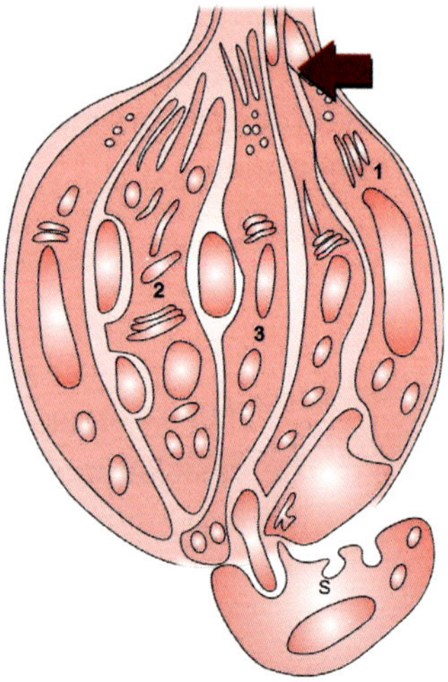

Fig. 6.1: Diagrammatic representation of a taste pore. 1, 2, 3 indicate type I, II and III cells respectively. S indicates type IV basal (sustentacular) cell

Dynamic Properties of Taste Bud

Taste bud cells undergo rapid cellular turnover. Autoradiographic techniques label the basal cells first, followed by type I and then, types III and II cells, respectively. These findings suggest that these cell types are transitional forms of a single cell line. The half-life of a taste bud cell is approximately 10 days. During turnover, the taste cells migrate from periphery to center of bud.

This dynamic nature of taste buds brings into focus the relationship of nerve fibers to a migrating taste cell.

One possible relationship is that taste bud cells are passed from one set of nerve endings to another during migration. This phenomenon can have a significant implication for the response stability of an afferent taste fiber. If fibers connect and reconnect during migration, the response of the afferent fibers will remain stable throughout their migration.

Another dynamic property of taste buds is regeneration. Damage to the gustatory nerve results in disappearance of taste buds, which then reappear following regeneration.

Central Taste Pathways

Central Termination of Gustatory Afferent Fibers

Gustatory afferent fibers from the Facial (VII), Glossopharyngeal (IX) and Vagus (X) nerves terminate in a rostral to caudal sequence within the ipsilateral nucleus tractus solitarius. The cell bodies of the gustatory fibers of these three cranial nerves are situated in the geniculate, petrosal and nodose ganglia, respectively.

The central sensory branch of the facial nerve formed from the merger of the chorda tympani and greater petrosal nerves is composed entirely of gustatory fibers.

The central part of glossopharyngeal nerve contains both gustatory and somatosensory fibers. However, because the glossopharyngeal nerve innervates a large number of taste buds, the number of gustatory fibers in the glossopharyngeal projection is probably larger than in the facial projection.

The vagus nerve is the largest nerve terminating in the nucleus tractus solitarius, but only one branch, the superior laryngeal nerve, contains significant numbers of chemosensory fibers.

Axons of these three cranial nerves penetrate the lateral border of the medulla in fascicles and pass through the spinal trigeminal tract and nucleus, turning rostrally along the lateral border of nucleus tractus solitarius to form the solitary tract. Each descending fiber of the solitary tract gives off several collateral branches that enter the nucleus tractus solitarius to terminate on second order neurons.

References

1. Meyer J, Squier CA, Gerson SJ. In: The structure and function of oral mucosa. Pergamon Press, New York, 1984.
2. Robert M Bradley. Essentials of Oral Physiology. Harcourt Brace and company Asia Pvt. Ltd., Mosby USA.
3. Timothy S Miles, Birgitte Nauntofte, Peter Svensson. Clinical Oral Physiology. Quintessance Publishing Co. Ltd.

7

Olfaction

The sense of smell is important to all animals for food recognition, detection of predators, and prey and reproductive behaviour.

Olfactory Receptors

Olfactory receptors are located in two patches of mucosa on either side of nasal septum and are faint yellowish in color. The receptor patches are situated out of the main nasal air stream in the most superior part of nasal cavity. Odors reach the mucosa by airflow within nasal cavity.

Structure of Olfactory Mucosa

The olfactory mucosa is 100 to 200 μm thick and consists of an olfactory epithelium overlying the lamina propria.

Histologically, it has a pseudostratified columnar epithelium comprising of olfactory receptors, sustentacular (supporting) cells, and basal cells. The lamina propria contains bundles of olfactory receptor cell axons, Bowman's glands and blood vessels. The olfactory mucosa is covered by 35 μm-layered mucus secreted by sustentacular cells and Bowman's glands.

Olfactory receptor cells are bipolar neurons with cell bodies in the olfactory epithelium. A single small-diameter unmyelinated axon arises from the basal end of the soma of the olfactory receptor neuron, penetrates the basal lamina, and aggregates with other olfactory neuronal axons to form olfactory (I) cranial nerve.

A single dendrite extends from the apical end of the soma to the epithelial surface, terminating in an apical dendritic knob. Several motile cilia ranging in length from 20 to 200 μm, arise from the knob and extend into the overlying mucus layer. A second type of olfactory receptor with apical microvilli also exists. The olfactory epithelium contains high concentration of *olfactory marker protein*. This high molecular weight protein is found predominantly in olfactory neurons in their axons and dendrites. Besides olfactory marker protein, olfactory receptor cells, also contain, *carnosine*.

Olfactory receptor cells are separated from each other by columnar sustentacular cells that extend from the basal lamina of the epithelium to the epithelial surface.

Besides, providing mechanical support for the slender receptor neurons, sustentacular cells also contribute secretions to the olfactory mucous.

The supranuclear part of cell contains mucopolysaccharides that are released into the overlying mucous layer. Other functions suggested are:

1. Maintenance of an ionic reservoir for electrical activity of receptor neurons.
2. Uptake and transport of odorants.

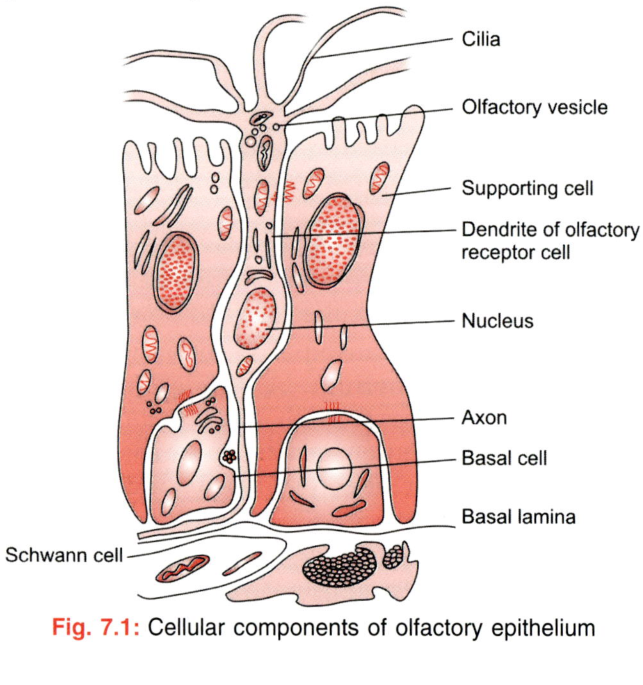

Fig. 7.1: Cellular components of olfactory epithelium

Prism-shaped basal cells are located close to the basal laminae arranged between basal ends of the sustentacular cells. Basal cells are progenitor cells that replenish the population of receptor mucous.

Dynamic Properties of Olfactory Neurons

Olfactory receptor neurons undergo continual renewal and are the only neurons in mature mammals to do so. Certain cells in the basal region of the epithelium function as progenitor cells. After mitosis, migration and maturation, they become functionally mature olfactory receptors.

Under normal conditions, an olfactory receptor neuron has a life span of 4 to 8 weeks, depending on the species. The senescent receptors are sloughed off from the surface of the epithelium to be replaced by newly formed receptor cells.

Receptor Mechanisms

The initial action in odor perception is the inhalation of a mixture of air and the odor. The odor molecules distribute over the epithelial receptor sheet as determined by the turbulence of the airflow, the shape of the nasal cavity, and the differential adsorption of the compounds with the mucosal surface. The odorant molecules with different chemical properties are distributed over the receptor sheet in an irregular pattern before any neural events take place.

Since the surface of olfactory mucosa is covered with mucus, odorants have to cross this layer to reach the olfactory receptors. The mucus layer moves across the surface of olfactory mucosa at 10 to 60 mm/minute toward the internal nares.

Therefore, the sequence of events taking place during odorant passage to receptors are:

1. Differential sorption of the odorants across the mucosal surface.
2. Diffusion of the odorants to the receptor neurons.
3. Interactions of odorants with chemoreceptive membranes.

Mucus is an aqueous solution of electrolytes and proteins. Many odorants in air occur in low concentrations of hydrophobic molecules that must traverse the hydrophilic mucus layer. The access of hydrophobic odorants to the olfactory receptors is thought to be enhanced by an odorant binding protein. The olfactory binding protein increases the odorant concentration in mucus layer by binding and solubilizing hydrophobic odorants in the mucus layer, and therefore, in the environment of the olfactory receptors. Odorant binding protein may function to remove odorants from the receptor environment as well.

Once the odorants cross the mucus layer, they interact with the olfactory receptor neurons to begin the process of molecular detection, odorant discrimination and sensory transduction.

The interaction of an odorant with chemosensory membrane initiates a series of membrane events associated with sensory transduction and subsequent electrical changes. Most odorants bind reversibly to the receptor, which is essential in preventing continued olfactory stimulation once the odorant gets removed.

Binding of an odorant molecule to a receptor molecule activates a GTP binding protein or G protein, which modulates the activity of adenylate cyclase, an enzyme that produces the second messenger, cAMP.

cAMP activates cAMP-dependent protein kinase to cause phosphorylation of ion channel peptides, thereby opening ion channels to produce changes in membrane potential.

G-protein in other receptor systems, such as α-adrenergic receptor, link membrane spanning receptors with enzymes inside the cell. All of these receptors share certain amino acid sequences, and are members of a "superfamily" with seven transmembrane regions.

Central Olfactory Pathways

Central Termination of Olfactory Afferent Fibers

Axons of olfactory receptor neurons aggregate into bundles passing through cribriform plate foramina. These axons then distribute over the surface of olfactory bulb, a layered structure, which is the site of first synaptic interactions in the olfactory pathway.

These olfactory cortex is a region that receives direct axonal input from olfactory bulb. This projection has many divisions:

- Anterior olfactory nucleus
- Piriform cortex
- Olfactory tubercle
- Cortical surface area of amygdala
- Temporal entorhinal complex.

Olfactory information is sent from the olfactory cortex to several other parts of brain, including orbital neocortex, the mediodorsal and submedial nuclei of thalamus, lateral hypothalamus, and the limbic area such as amygdala and hippocampus.

The neocortical projections are very close to the gustatory cortical area, and it has been suggested that these two areas overlap and thus form the neurobiological substrate responsible for flavor.

Reference

1. Robert M Bradley. Essentials of oral physiology. Harcourt Brace and company Asia Pvt. Ltd., Mosby USA.

8

Mechanoreceptors

Mechanoreceptors, are defined as, receptors designed to respond to mechanical stimuli.

Functions

1. Transmission of information on food texture
2. Sensory feedback

Classification

There are two major classes of mechanoreceptors:

1. Rapidly adapting receptors
2. Slowly adapting receptors

These two major classes of mechanoreceptors have been defined by their neurophysiologic response to a controlled stimulus. The stimulus required is mechanical deformation of their receptive fields. Receptor responses during a phase of application and removal of stimulus, are called the dynamic phase of stimulus. Receptor responses during a steady application of the stimulus, are called the static phase of stimulus.

Mechanoreceptors that generate action potentials during the dynamic phase of stimulus application are called rapidly adapting receptors.

Mechanoreceptors that fire action potentials during the dynamic and static phases of stimulus application are called slowly adapting receptors.

These receptors are innervated by large-diameter, fast-conducting, myelinated Aα fibers. Within these two mechanoreceptors classes, several other subclasses can be distinguished based upon the response characteristics of the receptors.

Both rapidly acting and slowly acting receptors are subclassified into two types: RA I and RA II and SA I and SA II, respectively.

Meissner's Corpuscles

These RA1 mechanoreceptors consist of crosslaminated structure containing nerve endings forming a column. Collagen fibers between the laminae connect the corpuscle to the basement membrane of the epithelium.

Merkel Cells

These are SAI mechanoreceptors consisting of a modified epithelial cell associated with a plate or disc-like expansion of nerve fiber terminals. These cells contact the surrounding epithelium by means of desmosomal junctions.

Pacinian Corpuscles

These are RAII mechanoreceptors arranged in concentric layers of Schwann cell lamellae surrounding an axon terminal. The receptive field of RAI and SAI mechanoreceptors is small with high and relatively uniform sensitivity across the center of these receptive fields which declines rapidly at the edges. In contrast, the receptive field of RAII/SAII mechanoreceptors is large, with a central zone of maximal sensitivity that slowly declines with increasing distance from the center.

Periodontal Ligament Mechanoreceptors

Spatial arrangement of receptors determines the response characteristics of periodontal ligament. Four types of neural termination have been described:

1. *Free nerve endings:* These ramify in a tree like configuration. They are located at regular intervals along the root length. They originate from unmyelinated fibers and carry a Schwann cell envelope with processes projecting into the surrounding connective tissue.

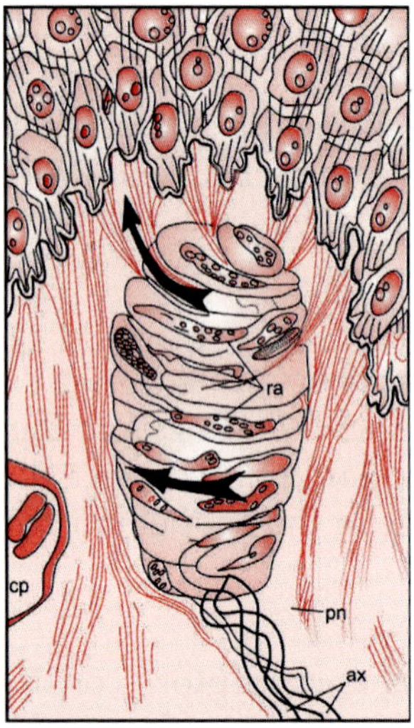

Fig. 8.1: Meissner's corpuscle: ax axon, pn peripheral nerve, ra rapidly acting receptors in cross-section, cp adjacent corpuscle

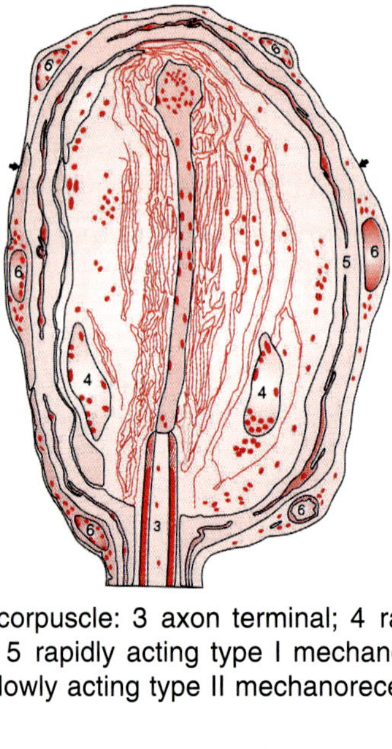

Fig. 8.2: Pacinian corpuscle: 3 axon terminal; 4 rapidly acting type II mechanoreceptors; 5 rapidly acting type I mechanoreceptor; 6 rapidly acting type II and slowly acting type II mechanoreceptors

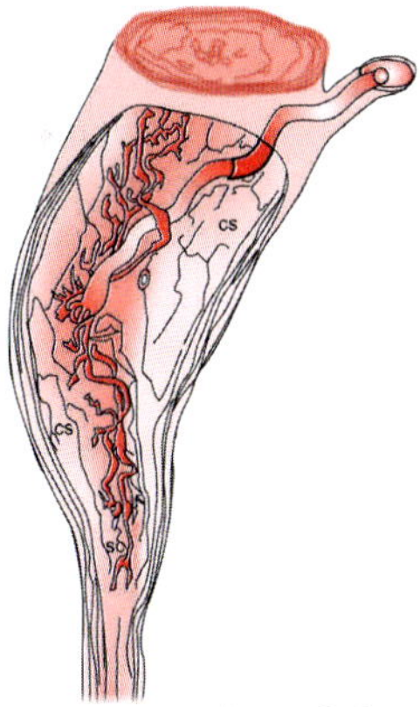

Fig. 8.3: Merkel cell: sc Schwann's cell; cs cross-section of mechano-receptor

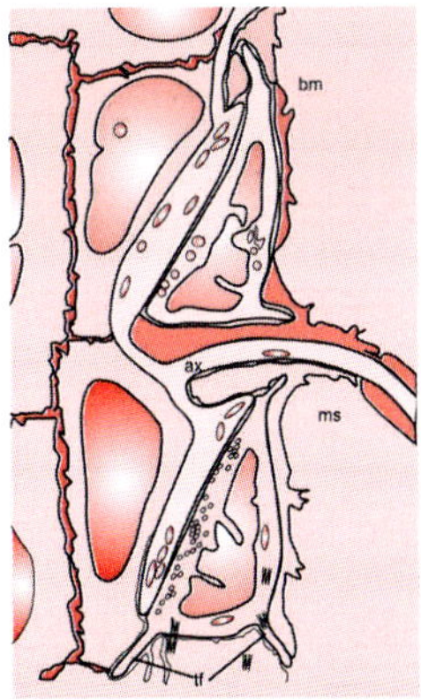

Fig. 8.4: Free nerve endings. ms muscle; bm basement membrane; ax axon; tf tanofilament

2. *Ruffini corpuscles:* These are found around the root apex. These are unencapsulated, dendritic and form terminal expansions among the periodontal ligament fiber bundles.
3. *Coiled form:* These are found in mid region of periodontal ligament.
4. *Spindle-like endings:* These are surrounded by a fibrous capsule and are found associated with the root apex.

Periodontal mechanoreceptors are innervated by afferent fibers with cell bodies in either trigeminal ganglion or the trigeminal mesencephalic nucleus. Both trigeminal and mesencephalic periodontal mechanoreceptors are distributed throughout the periodontal ligament. The mesencephalic mechanoreceptors are concentrated near the root apex while trigeminal mechanoreceptors are found around the middle of root.

References

1. Loescher AR, Robinson PP. Receptor characteristics of periodontal mechanosensitive units supplying the cat's lower canines. J of Neurophysiology 1989;62:971–78.
2. Lambrichts I, Creemers J, van Steenberghe D. Morphology of neural endings in the human periodontal ligament: an electron microscopic study. J Periodontal Res, 1992;27:199–o4.

9

Muscle Physiology

SKELETAL MUSCLES

Microscopic Anatomy of Skeletal Muscle

A typical skeletal muscle contains very long, cylindrical cells called *myofibers*. The muscle fibers are in parallel arrangement and range from 10 to 100 μm in diameter. The plasma membrane of a muscle cell is called a *sarcolemma* (sarco=flesh, lemma=sheath), whereas, the cytoplasm is termed as, *sarcoplasm*. Since the skeletal muscle arises from the fusion of numerous myoblasts during embryonic development, it comprises of numerous nuclei located at the periphery towards the sarcolemma. The mitochondria lie parallel throughout the muscle fibers, strategically close to the muscle proteins. The alternating light and dark bands of the myofibrils, give the muscle their characteristic cross-striations.

Myofibrils

Myofibrils are the contractile elements of skeletal muscle, which are 1–2 μm in diameter. They contain three types of myofilaments:

1. Thin filaments (8 mm diameter)
2. Thick filaments (16 mm diameter)
3. Elastic filaments

Depending on the contraction or relaxation of a fiber, the thick and thin filaments overlap over each other to varying degrees. The myofilaments are compartmentalized into *Sarcomeres* (sarco=flesh, meros=part) which form the basic functional unit of muscle fiber. Dense-appearing 'Z-lines' separate one sarcomere from another. Within each sarcomere, is a dense band called 'A or anisotropic band', comprising of thick filaments. The light or 'I or isotropic' band contains thin filaments. An 'H zone' is present in center of each of A band comprises of only thick filaments. H zone is divided in middle by 'M line', formed by myosin proteins.

MOLECULAR COMPOSITION

There are two contractile protein filaments in muscle:

a. Myosin

b. Actin.

Myosin Filaments

A myosin filament is composed of many myosin molecules (MW = 4,80,000). The myosin molecule is composed of six polypeptide chains:

1. *Heavy chains:* These are two in number, with MW = 2,00,000.
2. *Light chains:* These are four in number with MW = 20,000.

The two heavy chains wrap spirally around each other to form a double helix. One end of these heavy chains is folded into a *myosin head*. The elongated portion of the myosin molecule is called the *tail.* A part of the helical portion of each myosin molecule extends along the side forming *cross-bridges.* There are no cross-bridges heads in the very center of the myosin filament for about 0.2 μm since the hinged arms extend towards both ends of myosin filament away from the center. One of the important functions of myosin head is the *ATPase* activity. ATPase is required to breakdown ATP for utilization in contractile process.

Actin Filaments

The actin filament is composed of three proteins:

a. Actin

b. Tropomyosin

c. Troponin.

Actin

A double-stranded 'F-actin' protein molecule forms the backbone of actin filament. These strands are wound in a helical form with a complete revolution at every 70 nm. Each strand of the F-actin double helix is composed of polymerized G-actin molecules, each with a molecular weight of approximately 42,000. There are about thirteen G-actin molecules per revolution with an ADP molecule attached to each one of the G-actin molecule. These ADP molecules act as an active site on the actin filament with which cross-bridges of myosin molecules interact to cause muscle contraction.

Tropomyosin

Each tropomyosin molecule has a molecular weight of 70,000 and a length of 40 nm. These molecules are connected loosely with the F-actin strands, wrapped spirally around the sides of the F-actin helix. In the resting state, the tropomyosin molecules are believed to be on top of the active actin sites. Each tropomyosin molecule covers seven of these active sites.

Troponin

Troponin is a molecule present at one end of tropomyosin molecule. It is a complex of three loosely bound proteins:

a. Troponin I (Strong affinity for actin).

b. Troponin T (Affinity for Tropomyosin).

c. Troponin C (Affinity for calcium ions).

Elastic Filaments

An elastic filament is composed of a molecule, *titin* (*connectin*). Connectin is the third most abundant protein after actin and myosin. Titin anchors thick filaments to the Z discs, therefore, helping to stabilize the position of thick filaments. Its additional role is recovery of resting sarcomere length after muscle contraction or relaxation.

Types of Filaments in Skeletal Muscle Fibers

Filament	*Size and protein composition*	*Functions*
Thick	16 nm diameter, contains myosin (44%) bridges) move thin filament	Myosin heads (cross-filaments towards the center of a sarcomere during contraction.
Thin	8 nm diameter, contains actin (22%), troponin (5%), and tropomyosin (5%)	Contain myosin head binding sites; slides along thick filament during contraction.
Elastic	< 1 mm diameter, contains titin (connectin)	Anchors thick filament to Z discs and stabilize during contraction and relaxation.

A pure actin filament without the presence of troponin-tropomyosin complex binds strongly with the myosin heads in the presence of Mg^{2+} and ATP. If troponin-tropomyosin complex is added to the actin filament, the binding does not take place. Therefore, the active sites on an actin molecule of a relaxed muscle are inhibited by the troponin-tropomyosin complex which do not allow cause muscle contraction.

"Walk-Along" or "Ratchet" Theory of Contraction

Activation of actin filaments by calcium ions is followed by myosin heads' attachment to those active sites on actin filament. After the head attaches to an active site, changes in intramolecular forces between head and arm of the cross-bridges occurs. This new alignment causes the head to tilt towards the arm, thereby, dragging the actin filament along. This head tilt is called the *power stroke.*

Immediately following tilting, the head automatically breaks away the active site. Next, the head returns to its normal perpendicular position. It combines with a new active site, followed by a new power stroke moving the actin filament forward. Thus, the heads of the cross-bridges bend back and

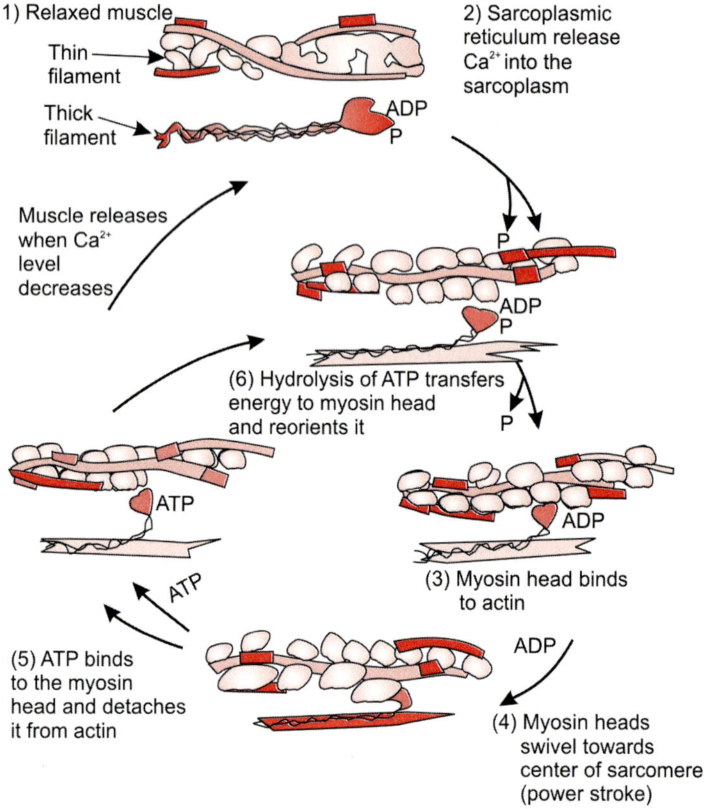

Fig. 9.1: Role of ATP in muscle contraction

forth and step-by-step walk along the actin filament, pulling the ends of the actin filaments towards the centre of myosin filament.

Masticatory muscles, in common with other skeletal muscles contain receptors known as *Golgi tendon organs*. These are located in the junction between muscle fibers and tendon. They are encapsulated sensory receptors through which a small bundle of muscle tendon fibers pass. The tendon organ has both dynamic and static responses, i.e. it responds rapidly when the muscle tension suddenly increases (dynamic response) but also settles down in a fraction of seconds settling down to a lower level of steady-state firing, i.e. directly proportional to muscle tension (static response).

References

1. Huxley AF, Gordon AM. Striation pattern in active and passive shortening of muscle. Nature 1962;193:280–84.
2. Janmey PA. Phosphoinositides and calcium as regulators of cellular actin assembly and disassembly. Annu Rev. Physiol 1994 ;56:169–72.
3. Schneider MF. Control of calcium release in functioning skeletal muscle fibers. Annu Rev. Physiol 1994;56:463–67.

10

Mastication and Deglutition

MASTICATION

The masticatory muscles are innervated by the motor branch of trigeminal (V cranial) nerve. Reticular formation stimulation near the brainstem centers for taste contributes towards mastication. Also, stimulation of areas in hypothalamus, amygdala and cerebral cortex near the sensory areas for taste and smell cause chewing.

Chewing Reflex

The presence of bolus causes or initiates reflex inhibition of masticatory muscles. This causes the jaw to drop. This drop, in turn, causes a stretch reflex of the jaw muscles leading to rebound contraction. This causes the jaw to rise and compress the bolus. This in turn, causes the inhibition of masticatory muscles, therefore, a cycle of repeated events.

DEGLUTITION

Deglutition or swallowing can be divided into:

1. *Voluntary stage:* Initiation of swallowing process.
2. *Pharyngeal stage:* Involuntary stage which constitutes passage of food through the pharynx into esophagus.
3. *Esophageal stage:* Involuntary stage that provides food passage to the stomach.

Voluntary Stage

The bolus, once ready, is passed posteriorly into the pharynx by upward and backward pressure of tongue against the palate.

Pharyngeal Stage

As the bolus enters the posterior mouth and pharynx, it causes stimulation of swallowing receptor areas all around the pharyngeal openings. Impulses from these areas pass to the brainstem thus, initiating a series of pharyngeal muscle contraction.

i. Soft palate pulls upward to close the posterior nares, thereby, preventing reflux of food into nasal cavities.
ii. Palatopharyngeal folds on either side of pharynx are pulled medially to approximate each other therefore, forming a slit through which food passes into the posterior pharynx.
iii. Laryngeal vocal folds become strongly approximated, and the larynx gets pulled upward and anteriorly by neck muscles. The epiglottis swings backwards, therefore, preventing passage of food into trachea.
iv. Laryngeal movement in upward direction opens up the esophageal opening. The upper 3 to 4 cm of the esophageal muscular wall, upper esophageal sphincter or pharyngo-esophageal sphincter relaxes thus, allowing food to move easily and freely from the posterior pharynx into the upper esophagus. This sphincter, between swallows, remains strongly contracted (as much as 60 mm Hg pressure in the esophageal lumen), thereby preventing air from going into esophagus during respiration.
v. At the same time, larynx is raised and the pharyngoesophageal sphincter is relaxed, the entire wall of pharynx contracts, beginning in the superior part and spreading downwards as a rapid peristaltic wave, propelling food into esophagus.

Nervous Control of Pharyngeal Phase

Impulses from posterior mouth and pharynx are transmitted through the sensory branches of the trigeminal and glossopharyngeal nerve into a region of medulla oblongata, *tractus solitarius*. The successive stages of swallowing process are controlled in sequence by neuronal areas of brainstem distributed throughout the reticular substance of medulla and lower portion of pons. The areas in medulla and lower pons that control swallowing, are collectively called, deglutition or swallowing center.

The motor impulses from the swallowing center to the pharynx and upper esophagus are transmitted by the 5th, 9th, 10th and 12th cervical nerves.

Esophageal Stage

The function of the esophagus is to conduct food from the pharynx to the stomach. The esophagus normally exhibits two types of peristaltic movements:

a. Primary peristalsis

b. Secondary peristalsis.

Primary peristalsis is a continuation of peristaltic wave beginning in pharynx and spreading into esophagus during the pharyngeal stage. Duration of passage is about 8 to 10 seconds.

Secondary peristalsis results from the distention of the esophagus by the retained food, which continue till all food empties into the stomach. Neural control of secondary peristalsis is by the esophageal myenteric nervous system and by vagal afferent fibers from esophagus to the medulla and back through vagal efferents.

INFANTILE SWALLOWING

There is a relatively high prevalence of anterior tongue positioning in children, which has been alternatively labeled as tongue thrust, deviate swallow, visceral or infantile swallow. Normally infants position the tongue anteriorly in mouth, at rest and during swallowing.

The first physiologic priority at birth is established of an airway so that respiration can begin. Accomplishment of this priority requires holding the tongue forward and down. An infant's normal swallow is characterized by strong lip activity to seize the nipple, placement of the tongue tip against the lower lip beneath the nipple, and relaxation of elevator muscles of the mandible so that the mouth open.

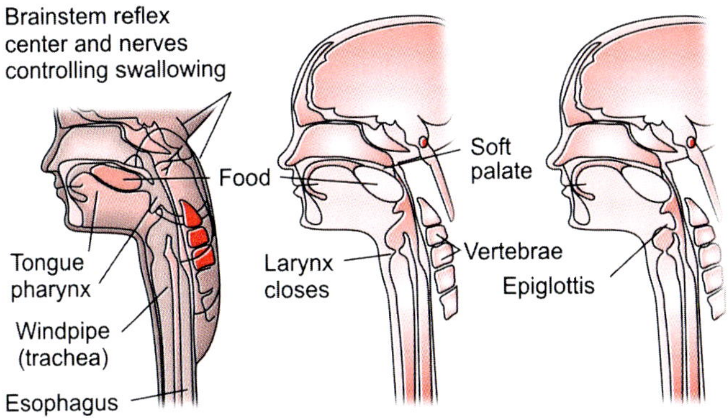

Fig. 10.1: Stages in swallowing

As oral function matures, there is a gradual activation of elevator muscles of mandible so that the mandible is brought upwards. Physiologic transition in swallowing begins during the first year of life and continues over next several years.

A mature swallow pattern is characterized by lip relaxation, placement of tongue behind maxillary incisors, and mandible elevation until posterior teeth contact.

References

1. Dean JA, McDonald RE, Avery DR. Management of the developing occlusion In: McDonald, Avery, Dean. Dentistry for the child and adolescent, 8th edition, Mosby, Missouri.
2. Graber JM, Vanarsdall RB, Vig KWL. Orthodontics. Current Principles and Techniques. 4th edition, Mosby, Missouri.

11 Dietary Influences on Oral Tissues

A balanced diet plays an important functional and maintenance role in oral environment and is constituted by–vitamins, fatty acids and minerals. Vitamins can be classified into:

1. *Fat-soluble vitamins:* Vitamin A, D, E and K.
2. *Water-soluble vitamins:* Vitamin B and C.

Required Daily Allowance (RDA) of Vitamins

A	50000 IU (International Unit)
Thiamine (B_1)	1.5 mg
Riboflavin (B_2)	1.8 mg
Niacin	20 mg
Ascorbic acid (C)	45 mg
D	400 IU
E (Tocopherol)	15 IU
K	70 μg
Folic acid (pteroyl glutamic acid)	0.4 mg
B_{12} (cobalamin)	3 μg
Pyridoxine	2 mg
Pantothenic acid	Unknown

Required Daily Allowance of Minerals

Sodium	3.0 gm
Potassium	1.0 gm
Chloride	3.5 gm
Calcium and phosphorus	1.2 gm

Iron	18.0 gm
Iodine	150 gm
Magnesium	0.4 gm
Cobalt, copper, manganese	Unknown
Zinc	15 mg

VITAMIN A

Beta-carotene: This is the precursor form of vitamin A.

Functions

a. It acts as an antioxidant and free radical scavenger.
b. It plays a role in immunomodulation.
c. It helps in increasing the numbers of T-helper and NK cells.
d. It inhibits mutagenesis.
e. Deficiency results in aberrant or increased keratinization due to inhibition of apoptosis and a resultant epidermal/epithelial differentiation.

Retinoids

Functions

a. Inhibit keratinization and terminal differentiation of epidermal cells.
b. Cell differentiation.
c. Antipromotion of DNA adducts.
d. Enhancement of cellular immunity.
e. Promotion of increase in synthesis/activity of TGF-β.
f. Arrest/reversal of leukoplakia progression.
g. Induction of cytotoxic and cytostatic effect on cancer cells.
h. Apoptosis.
i. Influence over DNA, RNA and gene expression.
j. Interference with carcinogenic stimulation/binding.
k. Antioxidant property.
l. Stimulation of tumor necrosis factor and epidermal growth factor activities.

Effect of Vitamin A Deficiency on Odontogenesis

The increased alveolar bone thickness can cut-off the vascular supply to the enamel organ thereby, resulting in its buckling, in parts or total degeneration. This causes the laying down of defective secretory products by the ameloblasts and the odontoblasts. The resultant effects of these changes are:

a. Enamel hypoplasia.
b. Irregular dentin deposition.
c. 'Cell inclusions' from pulp within dentin.
d. Wide predentin.

Effects on Oral Tissues

Vitamin A deficiency causes hyperplasia and keratinization of gingival, tongue and ductular system of salivary glands.

Role in Osseous Turnover

Vitamin A deficiency results in osteoclastic inactivity and increased activity of osteoblasts. This results in thickening of bone. This thickening of bone can cause a compression of nerves resulting in neural degeneration which is a feature of vitamin A deficiency.

VITAMIN E (α-TOCOPHEROL)

Functions

a. Free-radical scavenging.
b. Maintenance of membrane integrity.
c. Immune modulation.
d. Inhibition of cancer cell growth/differentiation.
e. Cytotoxicity.
f. Inhibition of mutagenesis and nitrosamine formation.
g. Synergistic action with selenium and vitamin C as an anti-oxidant.
h. Inhibition of DNA, RNA and protein synthesis in cancer cells.

VITAMIN D (EFFECTS ON TOOTH COMPONENTS)

Dentin

a. Widening of pre-dentin (indicating a delay in calcification).
b. Irregular interface between predentin and dentin.
c. Increased interglobular spaces.

Enamel

a. Faulty enamel matrix production.
b. Poor mineralization.
c. Irregular and pigmented enamel.

There is overall a hypoplasia of the tooth due to vitamin D deficiency.

VITAMIN K

Effect on Tooth Development

No changes/influences have been noted in vitamin K deficiency.

Effect on Oral Tissues

The most important oral manifestation is gingival bleeding. Hypovitaminosis K causes an impairment of fat absorption accompanied by obstructive jaundice, sprue and ulcerative colitis. Indirect liver involvement is the cause for increased gingival hemorrhage.

VITAMIN C

Functions

a. Antioxidant.
b. Reduce vitamin E degradation.
c. Enhancement of chemotaxis and phagocytosis.
d. Collagen synthesis.
e. Inhibition of nitrosamine formation.
f. Suppression of proto-oncogenes.
g. Enhancement of detoxification via cytochrome P450.

Effects of Ascorbate Deficiency in Tooth Components

Vitamin C deficiency causes atrophy and disorganization of the odontoblasts resulting in defective dentin deposition characterized by irregular dentinal tubules. Predentin is hypercalcified. Complete deficiency results in degeneration of enamel organ resulting in gaps in enamel deposition.

Effect on Alveolar Bone and Periodontal Ligament

In vitamin C deficiency, the osteoblasts revert to fibroblasts. This deficiency causes bone atrophy resulting in detachment of periodontal ligament fibers and subsequently, loosening of teeth.

VITAMIN B COMPLEX

Riboflavin Deficiency

The deficiency state of riboflavin manifests as:

a. Cheilosis
b. Angular stomatitis
c. Denudation of epithelium of lips causing redness.
d. Desquamation.
e. Glossitis due to enlargement and flattening of tips of papillae.

Vitamin B_1 (thiamine) Deficiency

B_1 deficiency manifests as marked sensitivity of oral mucosa and development of 'pin-point' vesicles on buccal mucosa, under the tongue and the palate.

Nicotinic Acid or Niacin Deficiency

The tongue becomes swollen, causing its pressing against the tooth surface resulting in indentations. Excessive salivation takes place. Gingiva becomes painful and is prone to infection.

Pantothenic Acid Deficiency

Pantothenic acid deficiency causes oral epithelial degeneration resulting in exposure of underlying connective tissue. Osteoporotic changes in alveolar bone are seen.

Pyridoxine (Vitamin B_6) Deficiency

Vitamin B_6 deficiency results in cheilosis, sore and swollen tongue.

Vitamin B_{12} Deficiency

Vitamin B_{12} deficiency manifests as pernicious anemia seen as soreness of tongue and painful ulcerations.

References

1. Baume LJ. Progressive atrophy and expulsion of upper rat incisor after prolonged vitamin A deficiency. J Dent Res 1969;48:330–35.
2. Fish EW, Harris LJ. The effects of vitamin C deficiency on tooth structures in guinea pigs. Brit Dent J 1935;58:3–6.
3. Oliver WM. Calcium deficiencies and collagen synthesis. J Periodontal Res 1969;7:29–35.
4. Euwonwu CO, Meeks VI. Bionutrition and oral cancer in humans. Crit Rev Oral Biol Med 1995;6(1):5–17.

Index

Reader's Notes

Reader's Notes

Reader's Notes

Reader's Notes

Reader's Notes